SpringerBriefs in Well-Being and Quality of Life Research

SpringerBriefs in Well-Being and Quality-of-Life Research are concise summaries of cutting-edge research and practical applications across the field of well-being and quality of life research. These compact refereed monographs are under the editorial supervision of an international Advisory Board*. Volumes are 50 to 125 pages (approximately 20,000–70,000 words), with a clear focus. The series covers a range of content from professional to academic such as: snapshots of hot and/or emerging topics, in-depth case studies, and timely reports of state-of-the art analytical techniques. The scope of the series spans the entire field of Well-Being Research and Quality-of-Life Studies, with a view to significantly advance research. The character of the series is international and interdisciplinary and will include research areas such as: health, cross-cultural studies, gender, children, education, work and organizational issues, relationships, job satisfaction, religion, spirituality, ageing from the perspectives of sociology, psychology, philosophy, public health and economics in relation to Well-being and Quality-of-Life research. Volumes in the series may analyze past, present and/or future trends, as well as their determinants and consequences. Both solicited and unsolicited manuscripts are considered for publication in this series. SpringerBriefs in Well-Being and Quality-of-Life Research will be of interest to a wide range of individuals with interest in quality of life studies, including sociologists, psychologists, economists, philosophers, health researchers, as well as practitioners across the social sciences. Briefs will be published as part of Springer's eBook collection, with millions of users worldwide. In addition, Briefs will be available for individual print and electronic purchase. Briefs are characterized by fast, global electronic dissemination, standard publishing contracts, easy-to-use manuscript preparation and formatting guidelines, and expedited production schedules. We aim for publication 8–12 weeks after acceptance. Both solicited and unsolicited manuscripts are considered for publication in this series.

More information about this series at http://www.springer.com/series/10150

Atefeh Ahmadi

Mindfulness Among Students

The Impact of Faculty and Demography in Malaysia

Springer

Atefeh Ahmadi
Faculty of Nursing and Midwifery
Kerman University of Medical Sciences
Kerman
Iran

ISSN 2211-7644 ISSN 2211-7652 (electronic)
SpringerBriefs in Well-Being and Quality of Life Research
ISBN 978-981-10-2780-2 ISBN 978-981-10-2781-9 (eBook)
DOI 10.1007/978-981-10-2781-9

Library of Congress Control Number: 2016953659

Printed on acid-free paper

This Springer imprint is published by Springer Nature
The registered company is Springer Nature Singapore Pte Ltd.
The registered company address is: 152 Beach Road, #22-06/08 Gateway East, Singapore 189721, Singapore

To my parents, husband and son for their undying support of my journey and their love and companionship along the way

Declaration

I declare that this book entitled: "Mindfulness Among Students: The Impact of Faculty and Demography in Malaysia" is the result of my own research except as cited in the references. The origin of this book has been accepted for my Master degree. I hereby declare that this work is an original research.

Preface

This study has been carried out to identify the level of mindfulness among undergraduate students in Universiti Teknologi Malaysia (UTM), Malaysia, and its relationship with their respective faculty as well as their unique demographic factors. A total of 273 first year, first semester students pursuing their bachelor degree in Education, Civil Engineering, Management, and Science were involved in this study. The questionnaire issued to them comprised of 15 items pertaining to the Mindfulness Attention Awareness Scale (MAAS) and eight items related to their individual characteristics. Analysis of the data has been done using "Statistical Package for Social Science" (SPSS version 19.0) where percentage and frequency were used in the descriptive analysis; bivariate-correlational analysis was done as the inferential analysis. The major finding of this study indicated that the students' average level of mindfulness, recorded at 3.77, was lower than the average score of the general population (3.86). The highest level of mindfulness was in the Faculty of Science (3.82) and the lowest was in the Faculty of Management (3.63). In addition, there was no relationship between the level of mindfulness and the type of faculty (a = 0.97). There was also no relationship between the level of mindfulness and age, gender, religion, race, educational background, and family condition. Nevertheless, there was a significant relationship between the level of mindfulness and health condition (a = 0.004). The implication, recommendation and limitation of the study were stated for practical application and future research.

Kerman, Iran Atefeh Ahmadi

Contents

Abbreviations

CAMS-R	The Cognitive Affective Mindfulness Scale-Revised
FFMQ	Five-Factor Mindfulness Questionnaire
FMI	The Freiburg Mindfulness Inventory
IAA model	Three Fundamental Components: Intention, Attention, and Attitude
KIMS	The Kentucky Inventory of Mindfulness Skills
MAAS	Mindfulness Attention Awareness Scale
SPSS	Statistical Package for Social Science
STAM	Sijil Tinggi Agama Malaysia
STPM	Sijil Tinggi Persekolahan Malaysia
TMS	The Toronto Mindfulness Scale
UTM	Universiti Teknologi Malaysia

List of Figures

List of Tables

Chapter 1
Introduction

Abstract Introduction of this chapter aimed to show what this research is about. Background of the study selected the most recent and most important studies about this area. Section three illustrated the importance of research, its benefits to others as well as lack of knowledge. In the following, research objectives, questions, and hypotheses consequently presented the goals of researcher to do the study, the questions that will be answered and null hypotheses before research about the objectives. Seventh part clarified the horizons and limits of the study. "Significance of the study" bolded the outcomes of the study for the beneficiaries of the research. The network of linked concepts and theories which are footstones of the topic are found, respectively, in conceptual framework and theoretical framework. Conceptual and operation definitions made the text easy to understand for who are not familiar with the dimensions of the research. In fact, conclusion showed what can be found out after reading all parts of this chapter.

Keywords Objectives · Framework · Problem statement

1.1 Introduction

Malaysia is aspired to achieve her year 2020 goal to become a developed country (Alavi and Mansor 2011). This means that the nurturing of more educated citizens with higher mental resilience is of major importance to drive development. In recent times, *Universiti Teknologi Malaysia* (UTM), the top engineering school in the country and a research university, has been rigorously conducting more research on mental hygiene, which includes the main topic of this research—mindfulness.

Change is an entity of life. People face challenges at every stage of life and this includes the stage where one attends university to pursue higher level of education. Most often than not, this major transition creates some psychological instabilities and reduce the mental hygiene to a certain extent. The background of the often young university student, i.e., his or her demographic factors, can have an influence

A. Ahmadi, *Mindfulness Among Students*, SpringerBriefs in Well-Being and Quality of Life Research, DOI 10.1007/978-981-10-2781-9_1

on the level of mental health. This is particularly true for his or her mindfulness which can ultimately affect his or her academic performance (Beauchemin et al. 2008) and social life not only in the present, but into his or her future.

Recent research in psychology and psychiatry has seen more attention given to the application of mindfulness to address mental health problems (Chiesa 2013). Mindfulness is a mental skill that helps to increase awareness and focused response of the mind to maladaptive behaviors and stresses (Bishop et al. 2004; Walach et al. 2006). It is the nonjudgmental awareness of external and internal daily moment–to-moment experience, rather than only related to external stimuli (Brown and Ryan 2003).

Having a mindful life decreases cognitive disturbance to reactive condition of mind that may increase emotional distress and continuation of psychopathology (Kabat-Zinn 1990). Management of stress and emotional problems and improvement of psychological well-being (Baer 2003, 2006a; Brown and Ryan 2003) that may include friendliness, acceptance, kindness, curiosity, and allowing (Segal et al. 2013) are the benefits of having a mindful life (Medvedev et al. 2016).

1.2 Background of Study

Entering the university as a fresh undergraduate student can be stressful because of the new environment which brings forth significant changes in social, financial, and often geographical conditions (Kawase et al. 2008). Furthermore, the student is often in his or her late teens, a stage where one may face some mental health issues (Lynch et al. 2011). In fact, some studies have confirmed that prevalence of mental and psychological illnesses tends to be higher among university students (Andrews and Wilding 2004; Lynch et al. 2011), which means that this is a group vulnerable to mental health deterioration.

Mindfulness, in the context of psychology, is the intentional use of awareness which includes compassionate and ethical inclination. Mindfulness is an understanding of what is occurring, before or beyond conceptual and emotional classifications about what is or has taken place (Brown et al. 2007). Furthermore, mindfulness has also been defined as a development of one's own memory (Chiesa 2013). Scientific research suggests that mindfulness and its practices have a significant impact on quality of life and health, encouraging psychologists to turn mindfulness into a mind-body practice to reduce the anxiety and stress, while at the same time promote well-being and coping skills (Crohn and Birnbaum 2010; Garland et al. 2011). This is in view that adaptive coping is a significant predictor to reduce anxiety, stress, and depression. Zimmaro et al. (2016) showed association of Dispositional Mindfulness with Stress, Cortisol, and Well-Being Among University Undergraduate Students.

Some studies have previously proposed systematic ways of cultivating mindfulness. These methods are currently being adapted for more efficacy and cost-effectiveness mindfulness practices to curb preventative self-care and health issues. Generally, mindfulness reduces stress while improving attention, immune function, saliva cortisol in group level, mood, and overall health. Mindfulness encourages meaningful interaction with the mind, body, and self to promote self-efficacy, problem focused coping, compassion, and satisfaction (Brausch 2011; Carlson et al. 2004; de Bruin et al. 2015; Dubert et al. 2016; Felton et al. 2015; Fuertes and Wayland 2015; Halland et al. 2015; Kuhlmann et al. 2015; Lynch et al. 2011; Matousek et al. 2010, 2011; Song and Lindquist 2015; Sudsuang et al. 1991; Van der Riet et al. 2015; Witek-Janusek et al. 2008).

Modern psychiatry has developed mindfulness-based therapeutic applications to enhance psychological quality and bring patient's attention to the present experience on a moment-to-moment basis (Marlatt and Kristeller 1999). Mindfulness has two components: The first one happens on immediate experience to self-regulation of attention for increasing recognition of mental events in the present moment. The second one is having enough orientation about experiences of the present moment. This awareness includes openness, acceptance, and curiosity (Bishop et al. 2004).

We can measure and evaluate the level of mindfulness by application of specified questionnaires. The most famous mindfulness instruments are the MAAS (the Mindfulness Attention Awareness Scale) (Brown and Ryan 2003), the Toronto Mindfulness Scale (Lau et al. 2006), and the Kentucky Inventory of Mindfulness Skills (Baer et al. 2004, 2006b).

Even though the universal qualities of attitudes cultivated in mindfulness such as nonjudgment, acceptance, patience, curiosity, and compassion are not linked to any particular population or condition (Morone and Greco 2014) but many factors may affect mindfulness, which include physical, mental, environmental, social factors, and so on. Demographic factors have profound influence, encouraging some studies to concentrate on the relationship between different demographic factors and their influence on mindfulness. The factors elucidated include gender, age, marital status, religion, race and nationality, and others. The relationship between nationality and mindfulness has also been studied, for instance, the study by the Elementary Education Online in 2012 revealed that the level of mindfulness among American students was significantly higher than Turkish students.

The present study focused more on demographic factors and these shall be discussed in details hereafter. In terms of gender, it is believed by some authors that mindfulness is one of the mind powers which is not governed by gender. For example, in a survey on Chinese students, partial factorial invariance across gender was shown (David et al. 2012). The relationship between mindfulness and religion seems to be close because according to the classical perspective on mindfulness, a degree of ethical judgment is necessary to the proper practice of mindfulness (Dhammika 1990). In fact, certain religions such as Buddhism promotes mindfulness at its core, but other religions also have different spectrum encouraging mindfulness. This is not influenced by any type of worship or any system of beliefs or statement of doctrine, any code of conduct nor any prescribed forms of ritual or religious observances (Ellis-Jones 2013). According to Baer et al. (2008), education and age are related to mindfulness because mind power and concentration are affected by one's brain power and spiritual levels. The relation between mindfulness and marriage, on the contrary, has fetched mixed comments. For instance, Frost (2012) stated that, "*Marriage has to be the greatest opportunity for mindfulness on the planet. Single, married and divorced people may have different level of mindfulness because having a spouse or not and even missing a spouse could effect on emotions and behaviors.*"

1.3 Statement of the Problem

The twenty-first century has seen some worrying level of mental health, particularly in the low level of mindfulness as a part of mental health. Having adequate mindfulness is necessary for attaining high achievement, not only in job, but also in daily life. Mindfulness is a key component of being a blissful human who has adequate consciousness and awareness in action and high quality of life (Ludwig and Kabat-Zinn 2008; Ruff and Elizabeth 2009). Mindfulness is a dynamic internal and experiential process which cannot be academically taught, but some demographic factors can be related to the lack or low level of mindfulness through their effects on the mind. A person's age, gender, marital status, religion, educational level, race, and nationality are some of these features.

A person's educational level can positively or negatively affect mindfulness. Receiving tertiary education can be a particularly stressful stage in a person's life because of the new environment and challenges it brings, such as new relationships and subjects; economical obstacles; new dormitories and disciplines; and anxiety about occupational future. These are often very different from a person's experiences in high school, suggesting that first-year undergraduate students are at the highest risk of mindlessness (Feldman et al. 2007). Trait mindfulness is negatively correlated with counterproductive academic behavior (Schwager et al. 2016). The faculty in which undergraduate students study, can have adverse effects on their mindfulness related to the contents of the courses. If the student is not well-prepared to take up the emotional, physical, and mental challenges, his or her mental hygiene can be jeopardized. There is no evidenced-based data about the current issues of mindfulness among tertiary students in Malaysia particularly at UTM.

In this research, the level of mindfulness among first-year undergraduate students was investigated. Furthermore, the relationship between the level of mindfulness and demographic factors of first-year undergraduate students, as well as its relation with faculties (Science Faculty, Education Faculty, Management Faculty, and Engineering Faculty) of Universiti Teknologi Malaysia (UTM) were investigated.

1.4 Research Objectives

The main objectives of this research were as follows:

1. To identify the level of mindfulness among first-year undergraduate students of UTM.
2. To identify the relationship between type of faculty and the level of mindfulness among first-year undergraduate students of UTM.
3. To identify the relationship between demographic factors and the level of mindfulness among first-year undergraduate students of UTM.

1.5 Research Questions

This study tried to answer the following questions:

1. What is the level of mindfulness among UTM first-year undergraduate students?
2. What is the relationship between the level of mindfulness among UTM first-year undergraduate students and type of faculty?
3. What is the relationship between the level of mindfulness and demographic factors among UTM first-year undergraduate students?

1.6 Research Hypotheses

The hypotheses posed in this study, corresponding to the research questions abovementioned, are as follows:

1. The level of mindfulness among UTM first-year undergraduate students is the same as the general population.
2. There is no relationship between type of faculty and the level of mindfulness among first-year undergraduate students of UTM.
3. There is no relationship between the level of mindfulness and demographic factors among first-year undergraduate students of UTM.

1.7 Scopes of Study

In order to quantitatively identify the level of mindfulness among first-year undergraduate students of UTM, Mindfulness Attention Awareness Scale was used. In addition, the students' demographic factors were gathered to find the relationship between the level of mindfulness and demographic factors of the students. The questionnaires distributed among students of four faculties of UTM (Faculty of Science, Faculty of Education, Faculty of Management, and Faculty of Civil Engineering) by cluster random sampling. The validity and reliability of the results are highly dependent on the trustworthiness and accuracy of the responses given.

1.8 Significance of Study

This quantitative study was done to identify the status of mindfulness among UTM first-year undergraduate students and the relationship between the level of mindfulness and demographic factors (age, gender, religion, family background, race, faculty, and health condition) of the students. The outcome of this study is significant in the sense where it assists the first-year students in achieving higher level of mental hygiene for better academic achievement and general well-being. With this, the students will have more positive energy. The results shall also help the academic institutions in formulating and promoting more programs that are beneficial to the students' mindfulness.

In addition to that, mindfulness has also been found to be a component addressed in counseling sessions and psychology clinics. Therefore, this research is beneficial to counselors and psychologists to better understand how mindfulness of undergraduate students is related to their demographic factors. All-in-all, the outcome of this study is deemed timely in addressing how mindfulness of undergraduate students can be possibly enhanced and understood better to help them in having better mental health which then propagates to their daily lives, academic performance, and future work places.

1.9 Conceptual Framework of Study

Figure 1.1 clearly illustrated the conceptual framework of the study formulated to achieve the research objectives. The sample of this study was the first-year undergraduate students from UTM who were, at the time of this study, in their first semester. The demographic specification (independent variables) in this research were: gender (male and female), age (17–21, 22–26, 27–31, 32 and above), religion (Islam, Christianity, Buddhism, Hindu, Irreligion, and others), race (Indian, Chinese, Malay, and others), family condition (live with both parents, single parent, or none of parents), health condition (having physical problems and/or psychological problems or none), educational background (matriculation, diploma, STPM/STAM, and others). The other independent variable of this study was the type of faculty (Education Faculty, Management Faculty, Science Faculty, and Civil Engineering Faculty). The questionnaire had 15 items in the Mindful Attention Awareness Scale (MAAS), each question had six categories.

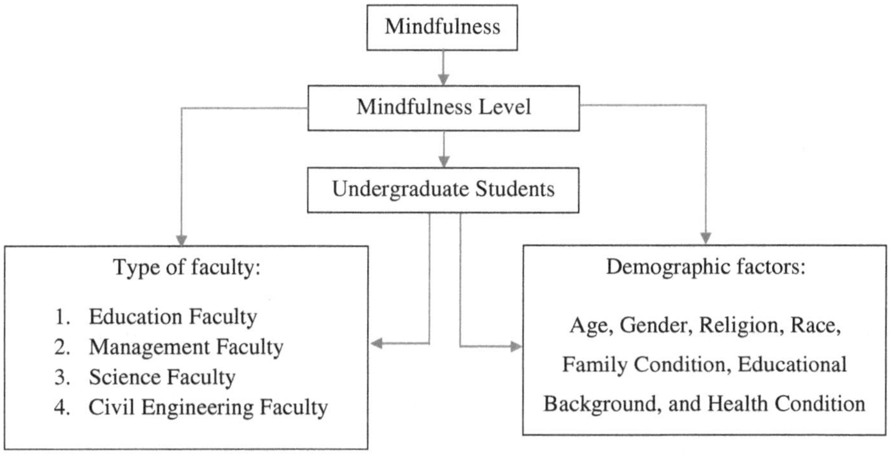

Fig. 1.1 Conceptual framework of the study

1.10 Theoretical Framework and Model of Mindfulness

A theoretical framework was formulated for this study to understand and organize the conceptual structure. This is a basic approach to perceive the issue of mindfulness systematically, and the application of theory allows structured interventions that will lead to positive changes in study (Gall and Borg 2003). This study utilized the Chaos theory and the Complex System Theory as the key theories.

Mindfulness is a multifaceted mental practice like the pieces of a mosaic. The four effects that it may bring include (a) better regulation of emotion, (b) focused attention, (c) greater awareness of the body, and (d) a changed perspective on the self. These shall be further elaborated hereafter.

The way one regulates emotions and deals with fearful threatening situations has a significant impact on self-sense. This can be enhanced through mindful practices that work as a versatile tool to facilitate everyday life's changes. If done through psychotherapy means, this can be done by increasing the felt senses of the body through different ways to increase one's sensitivity and awareness. A proposed theoretical model suggested emphasis on three aspects to increase mindfulness, i.e., intention, attitude, and attention (the IAA model). Intention is the basic reason to enhance mindfulness to change from self-regulation to self-exploration, and then to self-liberation over time. The ability to focus on a mental object, and also between objects, without thought processes is named "attention." Attitude refers to patience, compassion, patience, and acceptance of self-condemnation, which are the heart qualities of mindfulness (Shapiro et al. 2006). Mindfulness can also be improved through five facets: (a) observing experiences, (b) describing those experiences, (c) acting with awareness, and (d) and (e) nonjudgmental and nonreactive attitude toward inner experiences. From this, the Five-Factor Mindfulness Questionnaire (FFMQ) was created by Baer et al. (2006b).

Chaos is the change's science (Briggs and Peat 1999). This change does not happen in random, without structure, by formlessness, noise, and confusion, but it speaks of orders without constrained randomness and predictability. It is a shift to the belief in cause and effect after centuries of predicting, analyzing, and planning events (Wheatley 1999).

The chaos principles explicate the structure and behavior complexities of changes in chaotic systems: e.g., the weather, the movement of boiling water, and the patterns of arising smoke in windless environments. Changes cannot be easily predicted, even throughout existing science (Hutchinson and Smith 1996). Perhaps the most compelling aspect that the study of chaos has revealed is the relationship between order and disorder. Complex systems in chaos have the capacity to reorder themselves at a higher level of structural integration. Order can arise out of chaos and allow for adaptation, creativity, and self-renewal (Masterpasqua 1997).

Order and disorder are two sides of the same coin. A system experiences disorder moves to chaos, and out of that chaos evolves the next level of order. Our challenge is to embrace chaos in order to understand change, because "*It is hard to welcome disorder as a full partner in the search for order when we have expended such effort to bar it from the gates*" (Wheatley 1994). This challenge asks us to find ways of being that are contrary to Western culture. However, it is difficult for us to acknowledge that "*individuals most capable of adaptation and growth are those poised at the edge of chaos*" (Masterpasqua 1997). It asks a lot of us to know that "*it is necessary to disorganize before re-organizing.*" The reason being that 'stability and order' rather than 'disequilibrium, complexity, and chaos' have always been seen as hallmarks of well-being, but with chaos, one is opened up to new possibilities, to the unknown.

Mindfulness desires changing in mind to purposefully produce correct and true treatments in the present moment (Marlatt and Kristeller 1999). It involves a kind of non-elaborative nonjudgmental awareness; this attention-based thought, feeling, or sensation drives one to acknowledge and accept situations as it is. Such conscious awareness of one's current thoughts, feelings, and surroundings result in skills for controlling concentration, and is the first component of mindfulness often recognized as 'self-regulated attention.' The next component is one's orientation to mindfulness, which involves accepting one's mind stream; maintaining open and curious attitudes; and thinking in alternative categories (Bishop et al. 2004). Chaos means order without predictability, or constrained randomness and also construction of new, powerful, and nonjudgmental behavior.

1.11 Conceptual and Operational Definitions

This section shall explain the conceptual and operational definitions commonly found in this book. The conceptual definitions refer to those related to the elements of the research process in which a specific concept is defined as a measurable occurrence. The reader can gain a contextual understanding from the operational definitions which formed the foundation for this research in operational definitions.

UTM: UTM refers to Universiti Teknologi Malaysia. It is one of the popular universities in Malaysia in Johor (one of big province in Malaysia). The sample of this study was from UTM.

Mindfulness: Nonjudgmentally bringing one's full awareness to the present time and understanding manner, and having the ability to describe one's subjective experience and respond to it with intentionality (Baer 2006a; Baer et al. 2006b; Lau et al. 2006). Mindfulness is operationally defined in this study as the total scores of the Mindfulness Questionnaire.

Level: Level means an amount of something (Merriam-Webster Dictionary) and this research level has the same meaning to describe the amount or degree of mindfulness for each student. Mean of the scores of all students from the MAAS determined the level of mindfulness among the sample.

Impact: According to the Cambridge Dictionary it means a powerful effect that something, especially something new, has on a situation or a person. Here, it is the effect and the influence of faculty and demography on the level of mindfulness.

Race: Social interpretation of race is based on anatomical biological tagging in biology, and also social and cultural attributes (www.morebooks.de). In this study, it refers to the three common anatomic features in Malaysia, which are Malayan, Indian, and Chinese

Religion: Religion is a collection of belief and cultural systems toward the world view via symbols which relate humanity to the spiritually and moral values (Geertz 1973). In this study, religion means the collection of human belief to a superhuman with a controlling power (especially personal God/Gods) and worshiping Him. Here the common religions in Malaysia were identified based on the questionnaire responses.

Student: A student (also pupil) is a learner, or who attends an educational institution (Wikipedia). In this study, the people who are studying in first semester in four faculties of UTM (Science Faculty, Management Faculty, Education Faculty, and Civil Engineering Faculty) are research students.

Undergraduate: According to Harvey (2004), "*Undergraduate is a student who is undertaking a first-level degree program of study, normally a bachelor degree or equivalent.*" In this study, undergraduate means a student of UTM who has yet to receive a first degree and is studying to achieve first degree of the university.

Demographic Factors: These factors are a person's socioeconomic characteristics which can be shown statistically (e.g., sex, age, education level, occupation, income level, marital status, birth rate, death rate, and average age at marriage) (business dictionary). In this study, it refers to some characteristics such as gender, age, marital status, religion, faculty, race, and nationality of the UTM students in four faculties.

Faculty: A department or group of departments in a university (MACMILLAN Dictionary). In this study, it refers to fours departments in UTM, i.e., Science Faculty, Management Faculty, Education Faculty, and Civil Engineering Faculty.

STPM: The *Sijil Tinggi Persekolahan Malaysia* (Malaysian Higher School Certificate under the Ministry of Education) is one of the Malaysian preuniversity systems for admission to public universities.

STAM: *Sijil Tinggi Agama Malaysia* (Malaysian Higher Islamic Religious Certificate).

Matriculation: The Malaysian Matriculation Program under the Ministry of Education is a one or two-year preuniversity systems for admission to public universities. It is a race-based quota system.

1.12 Conclusion

This chapter presented a brief explanation of the research. University students represent a significant portion of a society which has an important in the development of the nation, and thus, their mental health is of great importance. Mindfulness is an important part of mental health that has been overlooked. The first three sections of this chapter show the importance of this research in the university and lack of studies in this area. This chapter has outlined the objectives of this study, which are to identify the relationship between certain demographic factors and mindfulness as well as its level among a group of undergraduate students in Malaysia. Theoretical and operational frameworks clarify theories that builded the context of this research as well as illustrating the way that research was done. Theoretical and operation definitions make the text easier to understanding for general population. The outcome of this study is deemed important for the respective authorities to formulate or promote activities which encourage mindful practices to have better mental health.

References

Alavi, M., & Mansor, S. M. S. (2011). Categories of problems among international students in Universiti Teknologi Malaysia. *Procedia-Social and Behavioral Sciences, 30*, 1581–1587

Andrews, B., & Wilding, J. M. (2004). The relation of depression and anxiety to life-stress and achievement in students. *British Journal of Psychology, 95*(4), 509–521.

Baer, R. (2003). Mindfulness training as a clinical intervention: A conceptual and empirical review. *Clinical Psychology: Science and Practice, 10*, 125–143.

Baer, R.A., (2006a). Mindfulness-Based Treatment Approaches: Clinician's Guide to Evidence Base and Applications. Academic Press, Burlington.

Baer, R., Smith, G., Hopkins, J., Krietemeyer, J., & Toney, L. (2006b). Using self-report assessment methods to explore facets of mindfulness. *Assessment, 13*(27–45), 61.

Baer, R. A., Smith, G. T., Lykins, E., Button, D., Krietemeyer, J., Sauer, S. … Williams, J. M. G. (2008). Construct validity of the five facet mindfulness questionnaire in meditating and non meditating samples. *Assessment, 15*(3), 329–342.

Beauchemin, J., Hutchins, T. L., & Fiona, P. (2008). Mindfulness meditation may lessen anxiety, promote social skills, and improve academic performance among adolescents with learning disabilities. *Journal of evidence based complementary and alternative medicine, 13*(1), 34–45.

Bishop, S., Lau, M., Shapiro, S., Carlson, L., Anderson, N., Carmody, J., et al. (2004). Mindfulness: A proposed operational definition. *Clinical Psychology: Science and Practice, 11* (3), 230–249.

Brausch, B. D. (2011). The role of mindfulness in academic stress, self-efficacy, and achievement in college students. Masters Theses. Paper 147. http://thekeep.eiu.edu/theses/147

Briggs, J., & Peat, F. D. (1999). *Seven life lessons of chaos: Timeless wisdom from the science of change.* New York: HarperCollins.

Brown, K. W., & Ryan, R. M. (2003). The benefits of being present: Mindfulness and its role in Psychological well-being. *Journal of Personality and Social Psychology, 84*(4), 822–848.

Brown, K. W., Ryan, R. M., & Creswell, J. D. (2007). Mindfulness: Theoretical foundations and evidence for its salutary effects. *Psychological Enquiry, 18*, 211–237.

Carlson, L. E., Speca, M., Patel, K. D., & Goodey, E. (2004). Mindfulness-based stress reduction in relation to quality of life, mood, symptoms of stress and levels of cortisol, dehydroepiandrosterone sulfate (DHEAS) and melatonin in breast and prostate cancer outpatients. *Psychoneuroendocrinology, 29*(4), 448–474.

Chiesa, A. (2013). The difficulty of defining mindfulness: Current thought and critical issues. *Mindfulness, 4*(3), 255–268.

Crohn, K., & Birnbaum, M. (2010). Environmental education evaluation: Time to reflect, time for change. *Evaluation and Program Planning, 32*(2), 155–158.

David, S., Sussman, S., Johnson, A., & Milam, J. (2012). Psychometric assessment of the mindful attention awareness scale (MAAS) among Chinese adolescents. *Assessment, 19*(1), 49–52.

de Bruin, E. I., Meppelink, R., & Bögels, S. M. (2015). Mindfulness in higher education: Awareness and attention in university students increase during and after participation in a mindfulness curriculum course. *Mindfulness, 6*(5), 1137–1142.

Dhammika, S. (1990). *All about Buddhism: A modern introduction to an ancient spiritual tradition.* Singapore: BDMS.

Dubert, C. J., Schumacher, A. M., Locker, L., Jr., Gutierrez, A. P., & Barnes, V. A. (2016). Mindfulness and emotion regulation among nursing students: Investigating the mediation effect of working memory capacity. *Mindfulness*, 1–10.

Ellis-Jones, I. (2013). Mindfulness and Islam. Retrieved 11 1, 2014, fromhttps://www.google.jo/gfe_rd=cr&ei=uSlVVPbUCe2q8wfejYHAAg#q=mindfulness+and+islam

Feldman, G., Hayes, A., Kumar, S., Greeson, J., & Laurenceau, J. (2007). Mindfulness and emotion regulation: The development and initial validation of the Cognitive and affective mindfulness scale-revised (CAMS-R). *Journal of Behavioral Assessment, 29*, 177–190.

Felton, T. M., Coates, L., & Christopher, J. C. (2015). Impact of mindfulness training on counseling students' perceptions of stress. *Mindfulness, 6*(2), 159–169.

Frost, M. T. (2012). Marrige. http://www.solveyourproblem.com/artman/publish/article_590.shtml

Fuertes, A., & Wayland, M. (2015, September). Cultivating mindfulness through meditation in a classroom setting from students' perspective. In *Innovations in Teaching and Learning Conference Proceedings* (Vol. 7, No. 1).

Gall, M. J., & Borg, W. (2003). *Educational research: An introduction* (7th ed.).

Garland, E. L., Gaylord, S. A., & Fredrickson, B. L. (2011). Positive reappraisal mediates the stress-reductive effects of mindfulness: An upward spiral process. *Mindfulness, 2*(1), 59–67.

Geertz, C. (1973). Religion as a cultural system (1973). In Basic Books. *Anthropological Approaches to the Study of Religion (pp.* 1-17). Psychology Press, Esfand.

Halland, E., de Vibe, M., Solhaug, I., Friborg, O., Rosenvinge, J. H., Tyssen, R. … Bjørndal, A. (2015). Mindfulness training improves problem-focused coping in psychology and medical students: results from a randomized controlled trial. *College Student Journal*, *49*(3), 387–398.

Hassan, A. (2006). Current practices of Malaysia higher education. *Globalization and Integration in Higher Education.*

Hutchinson, J., & Smith, A. D. (1996).Introduction. InN. Hutnik (Ed.), *Ethnicity* (pp. 3–16). Oxford, U.K.: Oxford University Press.

Kabat-Zinn, J. (1990). Full catastrophe living: Using the wisdom of your mind to face stress, pain and illness. Pain and illness

Kawase, E., Hashimoto, H., Sakamoto, H., Katsuki, Y., Iida, T., Umekage, R., et al. (2008). Variables associated with the need for support in mental health check-up of new undergraduate students. *Psychiatry and Clinical Neurosciences, 62*(1), 98–102.

Kuhlmann, S. M., Bürger, A., Esser, G., & Hammerle, F. (2015). A mindfulness-based stress prevention training for medical students (MediMind): Study protocol for a randomized controlled trial. *Trials, 16*(1), 1.

Lau, M. A., Bishop, S. R., Segal, Z. V., Buis, T., Anderson, N. D., Carlson, L., et al. (2006). The toronto mindfulness scale: Development and validation. *Clinical Psychology: Science and Practice, 62*(12), 1445–1467.

Ludwig, D. S., & Kabat-Zinn, J. (2008). Mindfulness in medicine. *American Medical Association, 300*(11), 1350–1352.

Lynch, S., Gander, M. L., Kohls, N., Kudielka, B., & Walach, H. (2011). Mindfulness based coping with university life: A non-randomized wait-list-controlled pilot evaluation. *Stress and Health, 27*(5), 365–375.

Marlatt, G. A., & Kristeller, J. L. (1999). Mindfulness and meditation. In W. R. Miller (Ed.), *Integrating spirituality into treatment: Resources for practitioners* (pp. 67–84).

Masterpasqua, F. (1997). Toward a dynamical developmental understanding of disorder. In *The psychological meaning of chaos: Translating theory into practice* (pp. 23–39). Washington, DC: American Psychological Association.

Matousek, R. H., Dobkin, P. L., & Pruessner, J. (2010). Cortisol as a marker for improvement in mindfulness-based stress reduction. *Complementary Therapies in Clinical Practice, 16*(1), 13–19. doi:10.1016/j.ctcp.2009.06.004.

Matousek, R. H., Pruessner, J. C., & Dobkin, P. L. (2011). Changes in the cortisol awakening response (car) following participation in mindfulness-based stress reduction in women who completed treatment for breast cancer. *Complementary Therapies in Clinical Practice, 17*(2), 65–70. doi:10.1016/j.ctcp.2010.10.005.

Medvedev, O. N., Siegert, R. J., Kersten, P., & Krägeloh, C. U. (2016). Rasch analysis of the Kentucky inventory of mindfulness skills. *Mindfulness*, 1–13.

Morone, N. E., & Greco, C. M. (2014). Adapting mindfulness meditation for the older adult. *Mindfulness, 5*(5), 610–612.

Ruff, M., & Elizabeth, R. (2009). The role of mindfulness in healthcare reform: A policy paper. *Mackenzie: Guest Editorial*, 313–323.

Schwager, I. T., Hülsheger, U. R., & Lang, J. W. (2016). Be aware to be on the square: Mindfulness and counterproductive academic behavior. *Personality and Individual Differences, 93*, 74–79.

Shapiro, S. L., Carlson, L. E., Astin, J. A., & Freedman, B. (2006). Mechanisms of mindfulness. *Journal of Clinical Psychology, 62*, 373–386.

Song, Y., & Lindquist, R. (2015). Effects of mindfulness-based stress reduction on depression, anxiety, stress and mindfulness in Korean nursing students. *Nurse Education Today, 35*(1), 86–90.

Sudsuang, R., Chentanez, V., & Veluvan, K. (1991). Effect of buddhist meditation on serum cortisol and total protein levels, blood pressure, pulse rate, lung volume and reaction time. *Physiology and Behavior, 50*(3), 543–548.

van der Riet, P., Rossiter, R., Kirby, D., Dluzewska, T., & Harmon, C. (2015). Piloting a stress management and mindfulness program for undergraduate nursing students: Student feedback and lessons learned. *Nurse Education Today, 35*(1), 44–49.

Walach, H., Buchheld, N., Buttenmüller, V., Kleinknecht, N., & Schmidt, S. (2006). Measuring mindfulness—the Freiburg mindfulness inventory (FMI). *Personality and Individual Differences, 40*, 1543–1555.

Wheatley, M. (1999). *Leadership and the new science.* CA: Berrellet-Koehler Publishers.

Witek-Janusek, L., Albuquerque, K., Chroniak, K. R., Chroniak, C., Durazo-Arvizu, R., & Mathews, H. L. (2008). Effect of mindfulness based stress reduction on immune function, quality of life and coping in women newly diagnosed with early stage breast cancer. *Brain, Behavior, and Immunity, 22*(6), 969–981.

Zimmaro, L. A., Salmon, P., Naidu, H., Rowe, J., Phillips, K., Rebholz, W. N. … Jablonski, M. E. (2016). Association of dispositional mindfulness with stress, cortisol, and well-being among university undergraduate students. *Mindfulness*, 1–12.

Chapter 2
Literature Review

Abstract Literature review is based on previous studies focused on similar objectives. Comparing the results of this study with them can support or violate their achievement. Definition and value of mindfulness as the main keypoint of the research and its relationship with population of the research as well as independent variables of the study were illustrated in this chapter. Famous standard instruments measuring mindfulness as well as which one used in this research were described. Characteristics of sample of this study were placed at the end of the chapter.

Keywords Mindfulness · University · Age · Gender · Religion · Educational level · Health condition · Race · Family status · MAAS

2.1 Introduction

There is a large body of published literature regarding the application of mindfulness to address a broad range of difficulties and the development qualities (Davis 2014). This chapter discusses recent studies on mindfulness with emphasis on those related to university students and demographic factors. Literature review shows the importance of a study based on the point of previous researchers view as well as lack of study in that area. The value of mindfulness in life shall be discussed accordingly and different definitions of mindfulness shall be put forth before the relationship between mindfulness and university students is discussed and linked to this study. Different ways of measuring mindfulness shall also be elucidated and a brief introduction to Universiti Teknologi Malaysia shall be given. This chapter shall conclude with a summary of the main points previously discussed.

A. Ahmadi, *Mindfulness Among Students*, SpringerBriefs in Well-Being and Quality of Life Research, DOI 10.1007/978-981-10-2781-9_2

2.2 The Value of Mindfulness in Life

Throughout their lives, most individuals encounter many challenging, and possibly traumatic, situations. How people respond to difficulties ranging from everyday problems to life threatening traumas determines how successfully they are able to cope with and overcome them. For example, although two people may have experienced the same difficult situation or environment, one person may cope effectively and seem to be minimally affected, or even positively influenced, while the other person may respond less effectively and experience less fulfillment or more psychological symptoms as a result (Collins 2009).

Sometimes we are swept away by the stream of thoughts, daily worries, psychological pressures and heavy responsibilities, and we prefer things to be different from what they are in this moment. This desire becomes stronger when we have pain and illness that further confound our attempts to feel better. Mindfulness can improve the quality of life by helping us to face the struggles we have in the experiences of life. So, the value and importance of mental health and mental power become utterly important here. Mindfulness is a part of mental hygiene which gives a person the coping ability to face challenging issues in life. In fact, mindful interventions have shown efficacy for a wide range of populations in treatment of psychological disorders (Baer 2003; Grossman et al. 2004; Hayes et al. 2006; Robins and Chapman 2004). In relation to this, mindfulness has found to be able to reduce social anxiety (Schmertz 2008).

Mindfulness increases moment to moment self-regulated behaviors; life satisfaction and well-being; human tolerance for logical approach; and acceptance of uncomfortable sensations and emotions (Eifert and Heffner 2003; Segal et al. 2003). Two components of self-regulating attention and adopting an open and accepting orientation toward one's experiences Mindfulness as the process of drawing novel distinctions or seeing things in new ways, help us to stay in the present (Langer and Moldoveanu 2000; Rempel 2012; Robins 2002). Mindfulness itself has been proposed as a measurable outcome of contemplative practices. Equanimity captures potentially the most important psychological element in the improvement of well-being (Desbordes et al. 2015).

Shapiro et al. (2006) considered three aspects for mindfulness: intention, attention, and attitude. It reduces the effects of negative psychological events, anxieties, depression, substance abuse, emotional instability, post-traumatic stress disorder, psychophysiological disorders, borderline personality disorder, and suicidal/self-harm behavior (Chiesa and Serretti 2011; Hofmann et al. 2010; Zoogman et al. 2015), and decreases recovery time after these events (Germer et al. 2005; Kabat-Zinn 1990; Shapiro et al. 2008). It makes balance in daily duties and enhances the awareness, control and openness in personal life to ultimately bring inner happiness (Shier and Graham 2011).

Mindfulness works on the cognitive part of brain with qualifying attention at the moment to improve the mind's flexibility in stressful conditions (Moore 2009). Just imagine, you are stuck in traffic, then now you realize that, in this unexpected situation, playing and speaking with your child riding with you is the best way not to waste your time and becoming frustrated or nervous (Wenk-Sormaz 2005). Mindfulness affects positive changes in self-regulation, values clarification, cognitive and behavioral flexibility, depression, rumination, stress, sleep quality and exposure (Caldwell et al. 2010; Carmody et al. 2009; McIndoo et al. 2016; Shapiro et al. 2006).

We need not react, think, or behave automatically as we always have done, dictated by thoughts, beliefs, and assumptions learned in the past. A mindful approach to experience is thus aligned with approaching experience with "a beginner's mind" (Bishop et al. 2004), which in turn fosters alternatives and creativity. Some well-documented benefits of mindfulness are as below:

1. Purposeful and self-regulated attention paid in a systematic way in the present moment (Marlatt and Kristeller 1999) combined with non-judgmental, multiple perspectives and conscious awareness that accept and acknowledge all thoughts, feelings, surroundings or sensation as the mind stream (Bishop et al. 2004; Silananda 1990).
2. Empowering skills for controlling concentration and having orientation to the moment by open and curious attitudes, and replacement of alternative categories, and as a whole coping with individual stresses, sufferings and problems (Grossman et al. 2004; Silananda 1990).
3. Ability to draw novel distinctions to create new perceptual categories, heightened sensitivity to the environment, and openness to new information (Demick 2000; Langer and Moldoveanu 2000).
4. Having appropriate insight by continual contact with experience. Subtle mind-full processes, like shining a flashlight inwards, to produce strong reactions and rapid change of mind stream (Laurie 2010).

On the contrary, mindlessness is characterized by the lack of attention to context due to reliance upon rigidly defined categories created in the past, and involves acting automatically without thought or knowledge of one's actions (Dauenhauer 2006) vice versa, in mindfulness. For instance, turning attention to breathing at any moment is intended to increase self-awareness and insight and reduces a maladaptive, automatic and habitual behaviors (Baer 2015). When thinking mindlessly, people may rely unquestioningly on information even if they have only been exposed to this information on one occasion or in one context that does not generalize to other situations (Demick 2000). Langer and Piper (1987) found that information presented in a mindful way leads to more creative use of novel objects than mindlessly presented information.

A significant point to note is that the concept of mindfulness has always been inclined towards spiritual movements rather than pure psychology. This has changed in the twentieth century where techniques associated with mindfulness were being applied in psychotherapy and this trend continued to expand in the early 1990s by integration of the discipline of mindfulness, originated from Buddhist roots, into clinical psychology as well as western philosophical systems (Sepp and

Embree 2010). In 2009, Langer empowered Western approach to mindfulness by proposing more creative and cognitive mindful approaches in psychology. Her view of mindfulness emphasizes on the openness to new data and perspectives, the increased control over the events of the moment, and devotion of more value to the process than the outcome.

Recently, academic research and studies about mindfulness, mindfulness-based interventions and its application in different organizations are increasing in Malaysia (Keng et al. 2015; Ling et al. 2015; Oly Ndubisi 2012) related to its positive impact integrating to psychological treatments, controlling and reducing cognitive and behavioral problems among different age groups, and promoting different aspects of mental health in social and individual life (e.g., stress reduction) (Hanan 2014; Hanan et al. 2011, 2013; Kar et al. 2014; King et al. 2011; Lan et al. 2014; Phang et al. 2016).

2.3 Mindfulness and University Students

Appropriate education needs self-mastery to deal with the responsibility required in today's world. Education is an area that often seems to abound in mindlessness (Langer and Moldoveanu 2000), but the potential for students to reap academic benefits from mindfulness is bountiful (www.ocbs.org). Research has confirmed that a college student's academic outcome is greatly influenced by his or her well-being. The term 'well-being' itself is a broad construct that can be defined in terms of theoretically and subjectively derived components characterized by hedonic (happiness and affect) and eudemonic (a sense of personal congruence in life) concepts (Karakashian 2011).

Mindfulness had direct relations with employee work well-being and employee's basic psychological needs at work. Autonomy support at work and work adjustment are affected by mindfulness. Mindful people were less likely to feel need frustration even in unsupportive managerial environment. Mindfulness thus appears to act as a protective factor in controlling work environments. These result highlights mindfulness as an indicator of wellness at the workplace (Schultz et al. 2015).

Researchers have shown students with higher well-being (included mindfulness) have better outcomes in relationships (Burger and Caldwell 2000; Cunningham et al. 1988; Lyubomirsky et al. 2005) and perform better on variables associated with improved college performance, such as flexible thinking, originality (Lyubomirsky et al. 2005), decreasing inter-cultural obstacles and engagement in pursuits that give them a boost throughout the semester (Nawiroh 2010; Sheldon and Lyubomirsky 2006). To date, some studies have documented a positive correlation between mindfulness and perceived health and psychological well-being, and a negative correlation with maladaptive aspects of perfectionism in college students (Perolini 2012).

The rationale for selecting college students to study on mindfulness is based on the unique challenges they have to negotiate at this developmental stage as well as the fact that, despite their young age, a high proportion of students endure physical and mental health problems. The period from the late teens through the mid-twenties has been recently termed ‘emerging adulthood’. This period is characterized by challenges related to identity exploration that emerging adults are expected to negotiate which bring about anxiety and uneasiness over the fact that several important areas of their lives are not yet settled (e.g., love, work and living arrangements). However, this period is also blessed with more freedom, limited structure, and world of possibilities (Arnett 2004; Kuhlmann et al. 2015; Song and Lindquist 2015; Van der Riet et al. 2015).

Changes of life in first year of university including pressure to get a good degree, relationship, academic and financial issues lead to worse results in measurement of mental health and wellbeing than general population and even than during their subsequent professional careers (Bonifas and Napoli 2014; Cooke et al. 2006; Monk 2004). Students with higher level of mindfulness have increased quality of life, ability to cope with the challenges of faculties, better engagement in activities, judgement and decision making, bloster stress management skills and better academic achievement (Bonifas and Napoli 2014; Karakashian 2011; Kurtz 2011; Leong and Rasli 2013; Leroy et al. 2013). Students who are mindful, either through their character or through learning, tend to experience greater well-being, and that being more mindful tends to accompany more positive emotion, greater popularity and having more friends, and less negative emotion and anxiety (Weare 2012).

The link between more mindful actions has also been made to the organizational environment where more rigid bureaucracies not only hinders a mindful condition, but also promotes a mindless standardization (Hoy and Tschannen-Moran 2003). This is against the nurturing of mindful students because they need an environment which encourages them to experiment more and not be frightened of making mistakes. This also means the nurturing of a culture of trust in which people are not afraid of breaking new ground, taking risks, and making errors. Weick and Sutcliffe (2011) opined that organizational mindfulness can be increased in five aspects, i.e., being prepared for defeat, sensitivity to quality, reluctance to simplify, being resilient, and greaten the expertise.

The notion promoted here is that mindfulness should be understood and practiced by administrators of academic settings. For example, the principals ought to encourage playing with ideas, creating novelty, producing safe environment to take reasonable risks. As the leaders of the institutions, they can have profound effects on school mindfulness (Hoy et al. 2006). Simply following the school rules with senseless orders makes teachers and administrators mindless. This also calls for more scrutiny and refinement of expectations; realization of the subtleties of the experiences; and creating novelty towards the administration of the institution to improve functioning and foresight (Hoy and Tschannen-Moran 2003; Langer and Piper 1987). All of these are to create mindful minds which have the vigilance, openness, flexibility, and the ability to break set. Overall, participation in a low-intensity mindfulness course in a university’s curriculum leads to an increased non-judgmental and non-reactive stance towards student’s thoughts, feelings, and emotions, during the course period, and their mindfulness increased even further after the course period. This increased mindfulness may help them in coping with stress given the pressure they are under and may improve their performance and their quality of life (De Bruin et al. 2015).

2.4 Mindfulness and Demographic Factors

This section shall elucidate the documented works on mindfulness and selective demographic factors, which include age, gender, race, education level, health condition, family status, and religion. More emphasis shall be given to the definition of mindfulness through different lenses of some major religions in this modern society as well as by irreligion.

2.4.1 Mindfulness and Age

Baer (2008) opined that age can have influence on mindfulness because age affects the mind's ability to concentrate and judge better. On the contrary, Lykins and Baer (2009) have shown that there is no relation between age and mindfulness in people who have or have not embarked on the journey towards higher mindfulness. Nevertheless, Eastern mindfulness meditation techniques have been found to have the ability to possibly postpone degenerating of chromosomes, which means helping the practitioner to stay younger and create greater subjective well-being. In addition, elderly practitioners seem to have more acceptance of their relative age (Park 2011). Schroevers and Brandsma (2010) found no relationship between mindfulness and age. Mindfulness appears to be a promising intervention modality for youth (Zoogman et al. 2015).

2.4.2 Mindfulness and Gender

McRae et al. (2008) believed that men respond better to cognitive regulation due to greater use of automatic emotion regulation. On the other hand, women use positive emotions during reappraising negative emotions more than men. Gender differences in stress responsiveness, adaptability, and level of mindfulness scores may be related to differences in sexual steroid concentrations, such as estrogens (Pico-Alfonso et al. 2007). In some other studies, marginal association was reported between gender and mindfulness with greater trait mindfulness in males (Cresswell et al. 2007). Schroevers and Brandsma (2010) and Bellinger et al. (2015) found no relationship between mindfulness and gender.

2.4.3 *Mindfulness and Race*

Bhui et al. (2008) found ethnic differences within religions. For example, they found that Black Caribbean Christians use more religious coping than Irish and White British Christians and that Bangladeshi Muslims showed more dependence on religious coping than Pakistani Muslims. On the same note, Bjorck et al. (2001) found that Christian Asian-Americans use religious coping more than Christian Caucasian-Americans. In comparing Asians versus all other ethnic groups, dispositional mindfulness is not necessarily associated with ethnicity (Cresswell et al. 2007).

2.4.4 *Mindfulness and Education Level*

In some previous studies, the educational level was not significantly associated with mindfulness (Schmertz 2008; Schroevers and Brandsma 2010) but Franco et al. (2010) saw that mindfulness had influence on the levels self-concept, academic performance, and anxiety. There are articles which investigated the relationship between mindfulness and student programs in the university. Most of the researches have investigated the relation between mindfulness mediation programs and levels of education, and concluded that education levels did not differ significantly between meditators and non-mediators (Lykins and Baer 2009).

2.4.5 *Mindfulness and Health Condition*

Mindfulness has relationship with positive psychological effects (subjective well-being and behavioral regulation) and negative correlation with psychological symptoms and emotional reactivity (Keng et al. 2011; Leary et al. 2006). Spiritual growth was positively correlated with post-traumatic growth, and the acceptance of events without judgment was negatively related with this growth (Chopko and Schwartz 2009). The elements of mindfulness reduce anxiety, psychological distress, rumination, fear, worry, and anger by promoting the skills to avoid, suppress, or over-engage distressing emotions and thoughts (Hayes and Feldman 2004; Kabat-Zinn 1990).

2.4.6 *Mindfulness and Family Status*

Mindful awareness in parenting interactions allows parents to shift their awareness to the present moment parenting experience. During long-term relationship with their child(ren), parents should attend to their child(ren)'s needs and exercise self-regulation to make wise choices in their actions towards the child(ren) (Duncan et al. 2009). Mindful parenting has been suggested to promote secure attachment relations between children and their parents (Siegel and Hartzell 2003). This has also been reported by Parent et al. (2011).

2.4.7 *Mindfulness and Religion*

Although mindfulness is based on Buddhist beliefs and practices, mindfulness principles are evident across a variety of belief systems and can be applied to many contexts (Wallace and Shapiro 2006). Religion is a cultural way of coping from which people derive meaning for their lives (Lhewak 2010). For example, Holroyd (2003) described mindfulness as a type of altered state and pointed out that it involves concentrating and letting thoughts go; this is practiced in several religions, including Christianity, Hinduism, and Judaism. In fact, the terms 'religion' and 'spirituality' are frequently used interchangeably in psychology research on coping (Bhui et al. 2008).

Koenig et al. (1998) defined 'religious coping' as the utilization of religious beliefs and behaviors in the process of solving problems and dealing with stressful life events. Others have defined it as coping that incorporates specific religious practices, identities, and knowledge (Bhui et al. 2008). Research has also shown that individuals who used positive religious coping strategies and religious tasks demonstrated greater positive psychological adjustment and well being (Baer 2015; Bosworth et al. 2003).

2.4.7.1 Islam

As the website www.mindfieldnortheast.co.uk has mentioned, "*Islam is largely a life-long pursuit of the mindful state. All men (and women) are expected to live their lives with the utmost awareness in each and every action, often going far beyond the requirements of 'holy men' and women in other faith systems, and every sphere of activity, vocational, domestic and evotional, is imbued with the same sanctity*". In line with this, researchers such as Loewenthal et al. (2001) have found that Muslims use more religious coping than non-Muslims.

2.4.7.2 Buddhism

Probably the oldest written reference to mindfulness is the notion of "Sati" in the Buddhist Pali canon (Schmidt 2011). As it is stated in www.buddhism.about.com, "*The Buddha taught people how to realize the enlightenment rather than teach doctrines of enlightenment. He believed the way we realize enlightenment is through direct experience and mindfulness without psychological barriers between the experience and human and also mental filters*".

Original Buddhist interpretation of mindfulness is "sustained, voluntary attention continuously focused on a familiar object without forgetting or distraction", interfering and meta-attention (monitoring one's own state of mind) (Grabovac et al. 2011; Thera 2014; Wallace and Shapiro 2006). A Buddhist's perspective on coping is that it is not just a reaction to stress, but also a way that one can be freed from suffering. Therefore, the goal is not to reduce the stress, but to change the individual's perspective or reaction to their stress through personal transformation using mental discipline (Chen 2006).

2.4.7.3 Christianity

"*All humans have been given the capacity of observing and grasping true and right concepts; it does not mean we take and practice a concept without critical thinking, but that we should be open to learn what our tradition has lost or ignored, or even deemed unnecessary to healthy life*" (www.Mindandsoul.info). This website also mentioned that "*Brother Lawrence found God present in whatever happened, or needed to be done, in the moment. He was choicelessly aware of the presence of his Lord in the sacredness of each moment*". It becomes clear at this point that mindfulness is within Christianity where God is believed to be present at the present moment.

2.4.7.4 Hinduism

In Hinduism, condition of calm consideration at the current present moment and condition of relaxed human mind, free of confusing feelings and thoughts are mentioned. The religion holds changing of the attitudes and encouraging religious enlightenment as the goals of Hindu Meditation. Based on this, two types of meditation have been born where one focuses on mindfulness meditation and another on concentrative meditation. In general, the mindfulness meditation is concerned on the experience and the perception of the human whereas the concentrative meditation focuses on the thoughtfulness on selected entities (www.radhasoamiji.org/hindu-meditation.htm).

2.4.7.5 Irreligion

For the non-religious, mindfulness is a power of mind not related to religion. It can help everyone to fulfill his or her psychological and physical deficits. In line with this, some modern scholars have encouraged religion to be kept as an 'identity' while mindfulness is taken as a kind of peace in our mental hygiene, acting separately from religious beliefs. Nevertheless, the association between mindfulness and religious practices continue to prove strong in leading changes in emotional states (Bhui et al. 2008).

2.5 Mindfulness Measurement

Consciousness consists of awareness and attention. Awareness is a continual background monitoring process and attention is a function of sensitively focusing awareness on the experience. Therefore, higher levels of mindfulness are equal to higher degrees of consciousness components (attention and awareness). However, there is substantial variability in these levels both within and between individuals (Black et al. 2012). A particular problem with mindfulness is the difficulty to observe and therefore to operationalize it. Even subjective information is challengeable since people who are not mindful do not recognize that they are not mindful (Eberth and Sedlmeier 2012). Trait and state of mindfulness have a wide spectrum (Mayer et al. 2011) with multidimensional constructs, as both are closely related but different constructs (Thompson and Waltz 2007).

There are eight currently available and validated mindfulness scales for adults (Bergomi et al. 2013) with intrinsically holistic with tightly interconnected aspects of mindfulness (Leary and Tate 2007). Some of them focus on specific populations such as clinical samples (Cognitive and Affective Mindfulness Scale, Southampton Mindfulness Questionnaire) or meditators (Freiburg Mindfulness Inventory).

- One of these is the Freiburg Mindfulness Inventory (FMI) (Buchheld et al. 2001; Walach et al. 2006) assessing openness to negative experience and non-judgemental present-moment observation. It was developed with mindfulness mediators.
- The Toronto Mindfulness Scale (TMS) (Lau et al. 2006) is often administered after a meditation exercise for the practitioners to rate the degree of awareness and accepting of their experiences during the meditation.
- In the Kentucky Inventory of Mindfulness Skills (KIMS) (Baer et al. 2004) measurement, four components of mindfulness are specified: accepting without judgment, describing, observing, and acting with awareness.
- The Five Facet Mindfulness Questionnaire (FFMQ) measures five factors of mindfulness (describing, observing, acting with awareness, no reactivity to inner experience, and non-judging of experience).
- The Southampton Mindfulness Questionnaire (SMQ) (Chadwick et al. 2008); first introduced as Mindfulness Questionnaire, MQ, Chadwick et al. (2005), unpublished manuscript, cited in Baer et al. (2006) is a 16-item scale with four related bipolar aspects of a mindful approach to distressing thoughts and images.

- The Cognitive Affective Mindfulness Scale—Revised (CAMS-R) (Feldman et al. 2007; Hayes and Feldman 2004) has a single factor construct of mindfulness with four components: orientation to present experience, awareness of experience, the regulation of attention, and acceptance/non-judgment towards experience.
- The Philadelphia Mindfulness Scale (PHLMS; Cardaciotto et al. 2008) is a 20-item questionnaire. The awareness subscale assesses noticing and being aware of thoughts, feelings, perceptions, and body sensations while the acceptance subscale is focused on the assessment of experiential avoidance.
- The Mindful Attention Awareness Scale (MAAS) (Brown and Ryan 2003) is a 15-item single factor self-report instrument measuring mindful trait. Attention to and awareness of life's experiences has been termed trait mindfulness. Day-to-day mindfulness or dispositional mindfulness is defined by Brown and Ryan (2003) as an inherent state of consciousness varying between and within a human that is characterized by the presence or absence of attention to or awareness of what is occurring in present experience.

The MAAS to be significantly and inversely associated, in medium-to-large magnitude, with a variety of mental health indicators (e.g., anxiety, hostility, depression, impulsiveness, somatization, disturbed mood, neuroticism, and negative affect) and positively associated with mental and physical health (e.g., self-esteem, optimism, positive affect, autonomy, self-control, perceived general health, physical functioning, and life satisfaction (Black et al. 2012).

Respondents rate how often they are preoccupied and not pay attention to the present moment and act on automatic decision. This questionnaire is rated on 6-point Likert-type scale ('almost always' to 'almost never') and scores are ranged from 15 to 90 and higher scores indicated higher level of mindfulness. It has good internal consistency (alphas of 0.87 and 0.82 in adult and student samples, respectively). Its validity has been adequate and has the capability to distinguish mindfulness practitioners from the general population (Brown and Ryan 2003; Höfling et al. 2011).

This instrument was chosen for this study among above questionnaires for using in academic setting among undergraduate students. It is a subjective instrument, easy to administer, available, and low time consuming to answer. Secondly, its English version is easy to understand for undergraduate students in the first semester that may have not good English language. In addition, mindfulness as measured by the scale is positively related to a variety of well-being constructs (Dundas et al. 2013). Lastly, some of the developed instruments are specified for clinical populations, often administered after a meditation exercise (The Toronto Mindfulness Scale), or are developed with mindfulness mediators (e.g., Freiburg Mindfulness Inventory) while MAAS has not this characteristics.

2.6 Students in Universiti Teknologi Malaysia

Universiti Teknologi Malaysia, literally translated into The Malaysian University of Technology, is one of the five public universities recognized by the Malaysian Government as the leading research and educational hub. Increasing the number of universities while expanding the number of courses and accepting more students each year is a governmental policy in Malaysia (Alavi and Mansor 2011). This is to produce the type of graduate that can share knowledge and global collaboration. In UTM, the number of both local and foreign students have been increasing every year where the number of international students reached 2324 in 2010 (www.sps.utm.my), coming from countries such as Indonesia, China, Iran, Pakistan, Maldives, India, Myanmar, Taiwan, Sri Lanka, and even as far as Belgium.

Based on Sovic (2009), international and also national students are disparate in groups of different experience, backgrounds, skills, and ages. Therefore, though they study in similar environment, their perceived experience and challenges may be different (Lee and Rice 2007). Langer and Moldoveanu (2000) argued that the ability of organisations to achieve reliable performance in a changing environment depends on how individuals think, gather information, perceive the environment around them, and whether they could change their perspective to reflect the situation at hand. These abilities can definitely improve university wellbeing.

There is a significant improvement in "Malaysian Wellbeing Index" from 2000 to 2012. It can be attributed to the wide range of policies and programmes that have been implemented by the Government to enhance the quality and standard of living (Unit 2013). Panahi, Yunus and Roslan in 2013 in a study about "Correlates of Psychological Well-being amongst Graduate Students in Malaysia" found there were significant differences in overall psychological well-being in terms of different faculties, age, semester of study, gender and marital status. However, there are no significant differences in psychological well-being of graduate students across different races and family sizes (Clark et al. 2014).

On the other hand, in the study of Clark and his colleagues significant differences between the male and female Malaysian students were noted with males rating their subjective wellbeing as higher than the ratings by females. The younger students rated their happiness as significantly higher on the majority of life domains. Those attending Chinese schools rated themselves substantially higher in regard to their happiness with "achievement in life" while those in the other schools rated themselves higher on most of the other domains as well as significantly higher on "satisfaction with life as a whole".

2.7 Conclusion

This chapter shall conclude here with some re-cap of the major discussion points. Practice of mindfulness has long been associated with religion, and in recent times, the promoting of mindful practices has been extended into psychology with no particular religion being mentioned. The value of mindfulness in life, alongside its different definition, shows that it is an integral part of mental health which has been studied, though not extensively. Stepping into university to pursue tertiary education is a major life turning point for many emerging adults, promising much hope but also stresses as they struggle to cope with the new environment; this has become the main reason for this study to select university students as the study sample.

The relationship between their demographic factors and level of mindfulness is of great interest, as some studies have documented significant relationship among the variables investigated. The discussion then proceeded to different ways of measuring mindfulness quantitatively. The discussion ended with a brief introduction to UTM as the leading research and educational hub in Malaysia and its composition of students.

References

Alavi, M., & Mansor, S. M. S. (2011). Categories of problems among international students in Universiti Teknologi Malaysia. *Procedia-Social and Behavioral Sciences, 30*, 1581–1587.

Arnett, J. (2004). *Emerging adulthood: The winding road from the late teens through the twenties*. USA: OUP.

Baer, R. (2003). Mindfulness training as a clinical intervention: A conceptual and empirical review. *Clinical Psychology: Science and Practice, 10*, 125–143.

Baer, R. (2008). Construct validity of the five facet mindfulness questionnaire in meditating and none meditating samples, *15*(3).

Baer, R. A. (Ed.). (2015). *Mindfulness-based treatment approaches: Clinician's guide to evidence base and applications*. Academic Press.

Baer, R. A., Smith, G. T., Hopkins, J., Krietemeyer, J., & Toney, L. (2006). Using self-report assessment methods to explore facets of mindfulness. *Assessment, 13*, 27–45.

Baer, R. A.., Smith, G. T., & Allen, K. B. (2004). Assessment of mindfulness by self-report the Kentucky inventory of mindfulness skills. *Assessment, 11*(3), 191–206.

Bellinger, D. B., DeCaro, M. S., & Ralston, P. A. (2015). Mindfulness, anxiety, and high-stakes mathematics performance in the laboratory and classroom. *Consciousness and Cognition, 37*, 123–132.

Bergomi, C., Tschacher, W., & Kupper, Z. (2013). The assessment of mindfulness with self-report measures: Existing scales and open issues. *Mindfulness, 4*(3), 191–202.

Bhui, K., King, M., Dein, S., & O'Connor, W. (2008). Ethnicity and religious coping with mental distress. *Journal of Mental Health, 17*(2), 141–151.

Bishop, S., Lau, M., Shapiro, S., Carlson, L., Anderson, N., Carmody, J., et al. (2004). Mindfulness: A proposed operational definition. *Clinical Psychology: Science and Practice, 11* (3), 230–249.

Bjorck, J., Cuthbertson, W., Thurman, J., & Lee, Y. S. (2001). Ethnicity, coping, and distress among Korean Americans, Filipino Americans, and Caucasian Americans. *Journal of Social Psychology, 141*, 421–442.

Black, D. S., Sussman, S., Johnson, C. A., & Milam, J. (2012). Psychometric assessment of the mindful attention awareness scale (MAAS) among Chinese adolescents. *Assessment, 19*(1), 42–52.

Bonifas, R. P., & Napoli, M. (2014). Mindfully increasing quality of life: A promising curriculum for MSW students. *Social Work Education, 33*(4), 469–484.

Bosworth, H., Park, K., McQuoid, D., Hays, J., & Steffens, D. (2003). The impact of religious practice and religious coping on geriatric depression. *International Journal of Geriatric Psychiatry, 18*, 905–914.

Brown, K. W., & Ryan, R. M. (2003). The benefits of being present: Mindfulness and its role in Psychological well-being. *Journal of Personality and Social Psychology, 84*(4), 822–848.

Buchheld, N., Grossman, P., & Walach, H. (2001). Measuring mindfulness in insight meditation (Vipassana) and meditation-based psychotherapy: The development of the Freiburg mindfulness inventory (FMI). *Journal for Meditation and Meditation Research, 1*, 11–34.

Burger, J. M., & Caldwell, D. F. (2000). Personality, social activities, job-search behavior and interview success: Distinguishing between PANAS trait positive affect and NEO extraversion. *Motivation and Emotion, 24*(1), 51–62.

Caldwell, K., Harrison, M., Adams, M., Quin, R. H., & Greeson, J. (2010). Developing mindfulness in college students through movement-based courses: Effects on self-regulatory self-efficacy, mood, stress, and sleep quality. *Journal of American College Health, 58*(5), 433–442.

Cardaciotto, L., Herbert, J. D., Forman, E. M., Moitra, E., & Farrow, V. (2008). The assessment of present-moment awareness and acceptance: The Philadelphia mindfulness scale. *Assessment, 15*, 204–223.

Carmody, J., Baer, R. A., Lykins, E. L. B., & Olendzki, N. (2009). An empirical study of the mechanisms of mindfulness in a mindfulness-based stress reduction program. *Journal of Clinical Psychology, 65*(6), 613–626.

Chadwick, P., Hember, M., Symes, J., Peters, E., Kuipers, E., & Dagnan, D. (2008). Responding mindfully to unpleasant thoughts and images: Reliability and validity of the Southampton mindfulness questionnaire (SMQ). *British Journal of Clinical Psychology, 47*, 451–455.

Chadwick, P., Hember, M., Mead, S., Lilley, B., & Dagnan, D. (2005). Responding mindfully to unpleasant thoughts and images: Reliability and validity of the Mindfulness Questionnaire. Unpublished manuscript, University of Southampton Royal South Hants Hospital, UK.

Chen, Y. (2006). Coping with suffering: The Buddhist perspective. *Handbook of multicultural perspectives on stress and coping*.

Chiesa, A., & Serretti, A. (2011). Mindfulness based cognitive therapy for psychiatric disorders: A systematic review and meta-analysis. *Psychiatry research, 187*(3), 441–453.

Chopko, B. A., & Schwartz, R. C. (2009). The relation between mindfulness and posttraumatic growth: A study of first responders to trauma-inducing incidents. *Mental Health Counseling, 31*(4), 363.

Clark, M., Amar-Singh, H. S., & Hashim, L. (2014). The subjective well-being of Malaysian school children: Grade level, gender and ethnicity. *Psychology*.

Collins, A. (2009). Life experiences and resilience in college students: A relationship influenced by hope and mindfulness (Doctoral dissertation, Texas A&M University).

Cooke, R., Bewick, B. M., Barkham, M., Bradley, M., & Audin, K. (2006). Measuring, monitoring and managing the psychological well-being of first year university students. *British Journal of Guidance & Counselling, 34*(4), 505–517.

Cresswell, D., David, C., Baldwin, M., Naomi, I., & Matthio, D. (2007). Neural correlates of dispositional mindfulness during affect labeling. *Psychosomatic Medicine, 69*, 560.

Cunningham, D. V., Van Tienhoven, A., & Gvaryahu, G. (1988). Population size, cage area, and dominance rank effects on productivity and well-being of laying hens. *Poultry Science, 67*(3), 399–406.

Dauenhauer, J. A. (2006). Mindfulness theory and professional family caregivers in longterm care facilities. *Journal of Aging Studies, 20*, 351–365.

Davis, T. S. (2014). A literature review exploring the potential of mindfulness as a tool to develop skills and qualities for effective consultation. *Mindfulness, 5*(6), 669–681.

De Bruin, E. I., Meppelink, R., & Bögels, S. M. (2015). Mindfulness in higher education: Awareness and attention in university students increase during and after participation in a mindfulness curriculum course. *Mindfulness, 6*(5), 1137–1142.

Demick, J. (2000). Toward a mindful psychological science: Theory and application. *Journal of Social Issues, 56*, 141–159.

Desbordes, G., Gard, T., Hoge, E. A., Hölzel, B. K., Kerr, C., Lazar, S. W., … & Vago, D. R. (2015). Moving beyond mindfulness: defining equanimity as an outcome measure in meditation and contemplative research. *Mindfulness*, *6*(2), 356–372.

Duncan, L. G., Coatsworth, J. D., & Greenberg, M. T. (2009). A model of mindful parenting: Implications for parent-child relationships and prevention research. *Clinical Child and Family Psychology Review, 12*(3), 255–270. doi:10.1007/s10567-009-0046-363

Dundas, I., Vøllestad, J., Binder, P. E., & Sivertsen, B. (2013). The five factor mindfulness questionnaire in Norway. *Scandinavian Journal of Psychology, 54*(3), 250–260.

Eberth, J., & Sedlmeier, P. (2012). The effects of mindfulness meditation: A meta-analysis. *Mindfulness, 3*(3), 174–189.

Eifert, G. H. & Heffner, M. (2003). The effects of acceptance versus control contexts on avoidance of panic-related symptoms. *Behavior Therapy and Experimental Psychiatry, 34*, 293.

Feldman, G., Hayes, A., Kumar, S., Greeson, J., & Laurenceau, J. (2007). Mindfulness and emotion regulation: The development and initial validation of the cognitive and affective mindfulness scale-revised (CAMS-R). *Journal of Behavioral Assessment, 29*, 177–190.

Franco, C., Mañas, I., Cangas, A., & Gallego, J. (2010). The applications of mindfulness with students of secondary school: Results on the academic performance. *Self-concept and Anxiety, 1*(3), 83–97.

Germer, C. K., Siegel, R., & Fulton, P. (2005). *Mindfulness and psychotherapy*. New York: Guilford Press.

Grabovac, A. D., Lau, M. A., & Willett, B. R. (2011). Mechanisms of mindfulness: A Buddhist psychological model. *Mindfulness*, *2*(3), 154–166.

Grossman, P., Neimann, L., Schmidt, S., & Walach, H. (2004). Mindfulness-based stress reduction and health benefits: A meta-analysis. *Psychosomatic Research, 57*, 35–43.

Hanan, S. A. (2014). An application of an extended theory of planned behaviour to understand drivers' compliance with the school zones speed limit in Australia and Malaysia.

Hanan, S. A., King, M. J., & Lewis, I. M. (2011). Understanding speeding in school zones in Malaysia and Australia using an extended theory of planned behaviour: The potential role of mindfulness. *Journal of the Australasian College of Road Safety, 22*(2), 56–62.

Hanan, S., King, M. J., & Lewis, I. M. (2013). Drivers' intention to comply with the speed limit in school zones, in Malaysia (Doctoral Dissertation, Queensland University of Technology).

Hayes, A. M., & Feldman, G. (2004). Clarifying the construct of mindfulness in the context of emotion regulation and the process of change in therapy. *Clinical Psychology: Science and Practice, 11*, 255–262.

Hayes, S. C., Luoma, J., Bond, F., Masuda, A., & Lillis, J. (2006). Acceptance and commitment therapy: Models, processes, and outcomes. *Behaviour Research and Therapy, 44*, 1–25.

Höfling, V., Moosbrugger, H., Schermelleh-Engel, K., & Heidenreich, T. (2011). Mindfulness or mindlessness? *European Journal of Psychological Assessment, 27*(1), 59–64.

Hofmann, S. G., Sawyer, A. T., Witt, A. A., & Oh, D. (2010). The effect of mindfulness-based therapy on anxiety and depression: A meta-analytic review. *Journal of Consulting and Clinical Psychology, 78*(2), 169–183.

Holroyd, J. (2003). The science of meditation and the state of hypnosis. *American Journal of Clinical Hypnosis*, *46*, 109–128.

Hoy, W. K., Gage, C. Q., & Tarter, C. J. (2006). School mindfulness and faculty trust: Necessary conditions for each other? *Educational Administration Quarterly, 42*(2), 236–255.

Hoy, W. K., & Tschannen-Moran, M. (2003). The conceptualization and measurement of faculty trust in schools: The omnibus t-scale. In W. K. Hoy & C. Miskel (Eds.), (pp. 181–208). 64.

Kabat-Zinn, J. (1990). Full catastrophe living: Using the wisdom of your mind to face stress, pain and illness. *Pain and Illness.*

Kar, P. C., Ling, K. S., & Chong, C. K. (2014). Mindful-STOP: Mindfulness made easy for stress reduction in medical students. *Education in Medicine Journal, 6*(2).

Karakashian, M. (2011). The predictive utility of mindfulness, experiential avoidance, and values-based action for well-being in college students. Doctoral Dissertation, The University of MEMPHIS.

Keng, S. L., Phang, C. K., & Oei, T. P. (2015). Effects of a brief mindfulness-based intervention program on psychological symptoms and well-being among medical students in Malaysia: A controlled study. *International Journal of Cognitive Therapy, 8*(4), 335–350.

Keng, S., Smoski, M. J., & Robins, C. J. (2011). Effects of mindfulness on psychological health: A review of empirical studies. *Clinical Psychology: Science & Practice*. doi:10.1016/j.cpr.2011.04.006

King, M. J., Lewis, I. M., & Abdul Hanan, S. (2011). Understanding speeding in school zones in Malaysia and Australia using an extended theory of planned behaviour: The potential role of mindfulness. *Journal of the Australasian College of Road Safety, 22*(2), 56.

Koenig, H. G., Pargament, K. I., & Nielsen, J. (1998). Religious coping and health status in medically ill hospitalized older adults. *Journal of Nervous and Mental Disease, 186*, 513–521.

Kuhlmann, S. M., Bürger, A., Esser, G., & Hammerle, F. (2015). A mindfulness-based stress prevention training for medical students (MediMind): Study protocol for a randomized controlled trial. *Trials, 16*(1), 1.

Kurtz, J. L. (2011). Happiness and self-knowledge: A positive psychology and judgment and decision-making hybrid course. *The Journal of Positive Psychology, 6*(6), 463–467.

Lan, H. K., Subramanian, P., Rahmat, N., & Kar, P. C. (2014). The effects of mindfulness training program on reducing stress and promoting well-being among nurses in critical care units. *Australian Journal of Advanced Nursing, The, 31*(3), 22.

Langer, E. J., & Moldoveanu, M. (2000). The construct of mindfulness. *Journal of Social Issues, 56*(1), 1–9.

Langer, E. J., & Piper, A. I. (1987). The prevention of mindlessness. *Personality and Social Psychology, 53*, 280–287.

Lau, M. A., Bishop, S. R., Segal, Z. V., Buis, T., Anderson, N. D., Carlson, L., et al. (2006). The Toronto mindfulness scale: Development and validation. *Clinical Psychology: Science & Practice, 62*(12), 1445–1467.

Laurie, H. K. C. (2010). Mindfulness, self-compassion, and happiness in non-meditators: A theoretical and empirical examination. *Personality and Individual Differences, 52*(202–227), 65.

Leary, M. R., Adams, C., & Tate, E. B. (2006). Hypo-egoic self-regulation: Exercising self-control by diminishing the influence of the self. *Journal of Personality, 74*(6), 1803–1832.

Leary, M. R., & Tate, E. B. (2007). The multi-faceted nature of mindfulness. *Psychological Inquiry, 18*, 251–255.

Lee, J., & Rice, C. (2007). Welcome to America? International student perceptions of discrimination. *Higher Education, 53*(3), 381–409.

Leong, C. T., & Rasli, A. (2013). Investigation of the Langer's mindfulness scale from an industry perspective and an examination of the relationship between the variables. *American Journal of Economics, 3*(5C), 74–81.

Leroy, H., Anseel, F., Dimitrova, N. G., & Sels, L. (2013). Mindfulness, authentic functioning, and work engagement: A growth modeling approach. *Journal of Vocational Behavior, 82*(3), 238–247.

Lhewak, D. (2010). Coping and distress among Tibetan survivors of torture and refugee trauma. Doctoral Dissertation, Boston University.

Loewenthal, K. M., Cinnirella, M., Evdoka, G., & Murphy, P. (2001). Faith conquers all? Beliefs about the role of religious factors in coping with depression among different cultural-religious groups in the UK. *British Journal of Medical Psychology, 74*(3), 293–303.

Ling, T. P., Noor, S. M., & Mustafa, H. (2015). Promoting interpretation through the concept of mindfulness: The case of selected heritage sites in Malaysia. *Advances in Environmental Biology*, 69–72.

Lykins, E. L., & Baer, R. A. (2009). Psychological functioning in a sample of long-term practitioners of mindfulness meditation. *Journal of Cognitive Psychotherapy, 23*(3), 226–241.

Lyubomirsky, S., King, L., & Diener, E. (2005). The benefits of frequent positive affect: Does happiness lead to success? *Psychological Bulletin, 131*(6), 803.

Marlatt, G. A., & Kristeller, J. L. (1999). Mindfulness and meditation. In W. R. Miller (Ed.), *Integrating spirituality into treatment: Resources for practitioners* (pp. 67–84).

Mayer, J. D., Roberts, R. D. & Barsade, S. G. (2011). Mindfulness, subjective well-being, and social work: Insight into their interconnection from social work practitioners, social work education. *The International Journal, 30*(1), 29–44, 66.

McIndoo, C. C., File, A. A., Preddy, T., Clark, C. G., & Hopko, D. R. (2016). Mindfulness-based therapy and behavioral activation: A randomized controlled trial with depressed college students. *Behaviour Research and Therapy, 77*, 118–128.

McRae, K., Ochsner, K. N., Mauss, I. B., Gabrieli, J. J., & Gross, J. J. (2008). Gender differences in emotion regulation: An fMRI study of cognitive reappraisal. *Group Processes & Intergroup Relations, 11*(2), 143–162.

Monk, E. (2004). Student mental health. Part 2: The main study and reflections of significant issues. *Counselling Psychology Quarterly, 17*, 33–43.

Moore, A. M. (2009). Meditation, mindfulness and cognitive flexibility. Liverpool John Moores University, School of Psychology, Liverpool, United Kingdom. *18*(1), 176–186.

Oly Ndubisi, N. (2012). Relationship quality: Upshot of mindfulness-based marketing strategy in small organisations. *International Journal of Quality & Reliability Management, 29*(6), 626–641.

Nawiroh, V. (2010). Mindfulness concept as solution to decrease inter-cultural communication obstacles: Case study of social interaction among Indonesian and Malaysian people. *Journal of Human Capital Development, 3*(1), 55–68.

Parent, J., Garai, E., Forehand, R., Potts, E. R., Haker, K., Champion, J. E., et al. (2011). Parent mindfulness and child outcome: The roles of parent depressive symptoms and parenting. *PMC*. doi:10.1007/s12671-010-0034-1

Park, J. S. (2011). The effects of perceived age, religiosity, and spirituality on subjective well-being in middle and later life. Doctoral Dissertation, State University of New York at Albany.

Perolini, P. (2012). Mindfulness and perfectionism as predictors of physical and psychological well-being in college students. ETD Collection for Fordham University. Paper AAI3461892. http://fordham.bepress.com/dissertations/AAI3461892

Phang, C. K., Chiang, K. C., Ng, L. O., Keng, S. L., & Oei, T. P. S. (2016). Effects of brief group mindfulness-based cognitive therapy for stress reduction among medical students in a Malaysian university. *Mindfulness, 7*(1), 189–197.

Pico-Alfonso, A., Mastorci, F., Ceresini, G., Ceda, M., Ghi, M., Pino, O., et al. (2007). Acute psychosocial challenge and cardiac autonomic response in women: The role of estrogens, corticosteroids, and behavioral coping styles. *Psychoneuroendocrinology, 32*, 451–463.

Rempel, K. D. (2012). Mindfulness for children and youth: a review of the literature with an argument for school-based implementation/Méditation de pleine conscience pour les enfants et les jeunes: Survol de la littérature et argumentation pour sa mise en oeuvre en milieu scolaire. *Canadian Journal of Counselling and Psychotherapy (Online), 46*(3), 201.

Robins, C. J. (2002). Zen principles and mindfulness practice in dialectical behavior therapy. *Cognitive and Behavioral Practice, 9*, 50–57.

Robins, C. J., & Chapman, A. L. (2004). Dialectical behavior therapy: Current status, recent developments, and future directions. *Personality Disorders, 18*, 73–89.

Schmertz, S. K. (2008). Rumination as a mediator of the relation between mindfulness and social anxiety in a clinical sample. Dissertation, Georgia State University.

Schmidt, S. (2011). Mindfulness in east and west–is it the same?. In *Neuroscience, consciousness and spirituality* (pp. 23–38). Netherlands: Springer.

Schroevers, M. J., & Brandsma, R. (2010). Is learning mindfulness associated with improved affect after mindfulness-based cognitive therapy? *British Journal of Psychology, 101*(1), 95–107.

Schultz, P. P., Ryan, R. M., Niemiec, C. P., Legate, N., & Williams, G. C. (2015). Mindfulness, work climate, and psychological need satisfaction in employee well-being. *Mindfulness, 6*(5), 971–985.

Sepp, H. R., & Embree, L. (Eds.). (2010). *Handbook of phenomenological aesthetics* (Vol. 59). Springer.

Shapiro, S. L., Carlson, L. E., Astin, J. A., & Freedman, B. (2006). Mechanisms of mindfulness. *Journal of Clinical Psychology, 62*, 373–386.

Shapiro, S., Oman, D., Thoresen, C., Plante, T., & Flinders, T. (2008). Cultivating mindfulness: Effects on well-being. *Clinical Psychology: Science & Practice, 64*(840–862), 67.

Sheldon, K. M., & Lyubomirsky, S. (2006). Achieving sustainable gains in happiness: Change your actions, not your circumstances. *Journal of Happiness Studies, 7*(1), 55–86.

Shier, M. L., & Graham, J. R. (2011). Mindfulness, subjective well-being, and social work: Insight into their interconnection from social work practitioners. *Social Work Education, 30*(1), 29–44.

Siegel, D. J., & Hartzell, M. (2003). *Parenting from the inside out: How a deeper self-understanding can help you raise children who thrive*. New York: Penguin.

Silananda, U. (1990). *Four foundations of mindfulness*. Boston: Wisdom Publications.

Song, Y., & Lindquist, R. (2015). Effects of mindfulness-based stress reduction on depression, anxiety, stress and mindfulness in Korean nursing students. *Nurse Education Today, 35*(1), 86–90.

Sovic, S. (2009). Hi-bye friends and the herd instinct: International and home students in the creative arts. *Higher Education, 58*(6), 747–761.

Thera, N. (2014). *The heart of Buddhist meditation: The Buddha's way of mindfulness*. Weiser Books.

Thompson, B. L., & Waltz, J. (2007). Everyday mindfulness and mindfulness meditation: Overlapping constructs or not? *Personality and Individual Differences, 43*, 1875–1885.

Unit, E. P. (2013). *Malaysian well-being report 2013*. Malaysia: Prime Minister's Department.

van der Riet, P., Rossiter, R., Kirby, D., Dluzewska, T., & Harmon, C. (2015). Piloting a stress management and mindfulness program for undergraduate nursing students: Student feedback and lessons learned. *Nurse Education Today, 35*(1), 44–49.

Wallace, B. A., & Shapiro, S. (2006). Mental balance and well-being: Building bridges between Buddhism and western psychology. *American Psychologist, 61*, 690–701.

Walach, H., Buchheld, N., Buttenmüller, V., Kleinknecht, N., & Schmidt, S. (2006). Measuring mindfulness—the Freiburg mindfulness inventory (FMI). *Personality and Individual Differences, 40*, 1543–1555.

Weare, K. (2012). Evidence for the impact of mindfulness on children and young people. The Mindfulness in Schools Project in association with Mood Disorders Centre.

Weick, K. E., & Sutcliffe, K. M. (2011). *Managing the unexpected: Resilient performance in an age of uncertainty* (Vol. 8). John Wiley & Sons.

Wenk-Sormaz, H. (2005). Meditation can reduce habitual responding. *Alternative Therapies, 11*, 42–58.

Zoogman, S., Goldberg, S. B., Hoyt, W. T., & Miller, L. (2015). Mindfulness interventions with youth: A meta-analysis. *Mindfulness, 6*(2), 290–302.

Chapter 3
Methodology

Abstract Design of the study is a guideline for the readers to show how the activities of the project are organized. Method of sampling show the scientific procedure was applied to access the final sample of the research. University Technology Malaysia was the location of the study. Socio-demographic factor as independent variable were part A and MASS was part B of the questionnaire. Research procedure systematically presented the consequent process of this study. Data process and analysis in this chapter described the screening part of data analysis.

Keywords Design · Sampling · Research location · Procedure · Data process

3.1 Introduction

Methodology is a set of organized procedures and guidelines which have been documented. It usually includes detailed explanation of patterns, techniques, frameworks, methods, and procedures applied to achieve the goals and objectives of the study. It is an important tool to guarantee the success of project. According to Thomas (2009), methodology is a study of methods that the research is going to use; it also explains why the research is using them. Research design addressed the procedures on data to access final outputs of the research; population and sampling show the informants of the study; research location is the local limitation of the research; instrument is the main tool used to access the data; research procedures briefly explain the steps from the decision for a study to final report of the whole research; data process and analyses approach mention the procedures from statical methods on the raw data used in this study to calculating final results based on the research objectives.

A. Ahmadi, *Mindfulness Among Students*, SpringerBriefs in Well-Being and Quality of Life Research, DOI 10.1007/978-981-10-2781-9_3

3.2 Research Design

The research design is a guideline for the researcher to be certain that the activities of the project are organized. According to Thomas (2009), research design is the plan which also takes into account the research expectations and the context. The main purpose of research is to solve problems, answer questions, and direct access to some relations. The answers may be gained through certain exploration, explanation, control, description, prediction, and practice (Sekaran 2003).

All aspects of a survey (from the establishment of a need for data to the production of final outputs including the micro data file, statistical series, and analysis) are described in the research design. This means that the design also addresses the pertaining statistics, population, execution time of research, accuracy, data collection, data analysis, sampling administrative, and operational and organizational issues.

This study used the method of a correlational research where variables are correlated with each other to find the relationship between them. Correlational research is usually used prior to experimentation or when experiments cannot be conducted for ethical or practical reasons. Quantitative measures had also been used to facilitate this correlational study to provide strong evidence for conclusion through corroboration and convergence of findings.

3.3 Population and the Sample

The sample of study is the group of research informants who provide the information needed for the study. A sample can make an inference about the performance of the large group (Gay et al. 2006). Sampling is important because it is a process to access research informants, but its size is dependent on the research methodology employed.

Random sampling was performed in this study where random first year undergraduate students from four faculties were taken to represent the entire population. This was done by firstly, stratifying all students to relatively homogeneous subgroups before segregating them to even smaller sample; this makes the analysis simpler, more balanced, and more economic. In addition, it is the best approach when the goal of the study is to compare the characteristics or behavior of people from different subgroups of sample. The four faculties involved were Education Faculty, Management Faculty, Science Faculty, and Civil Engineering Faculty. 272 undergraduate students were selected from 914 first semester students according to Krejcie and Morgan sample size Table 3.1.

Table 3.1 Sample size

No	Faculty	Population of first semester students	Selected percentage (%)	Sample
1	Education faculty	104	25	68
2	Science faculty	249	25	68
3	Management faculty	277	25	68
4	C. Engineering faculty	284	25	68
	Total	914	100	272

3.4 Research Location

University Technology Malaysia (UTM) is located in Skudai, a suburb of Johor Bahru city, Johor province, Malaysia. It is on of the biggest universities in Malaysia. Many national and international students study in this university.

3.5 Research Instrument

This study is an exploratory research using quantitative method. A questionnaire is a set of written questions tailored to get responses from all individuals in the sample group. It can contain open or close ended questions, and is a valuable as well as effective tool particularly when responses have to be gathered from a large number of populations. The structure of questionnaires is preferably simple with straightforward questions and no room for ambiguity. This can significantly reduce errors that can be made when interviews are being conducted and recorded. A questionnaire is also cost-effective, does not require verbal or eye contact, and its responses are not affected by the interviewer's mood or personal appearance (Gall et al. 2003). It was designed to answer the research questions using a short recommended scale (Grossman 2008, 2011) the Mindful Attention Awareness Scale (MAAS), developed by Brown and Ryan (2003) embedded in a customized questionnaire.

3.5.1 Research Questionnaire

Part A: This part seeks for the respondents' demographic information which includes gender, age, race, faculty, educational background, family status, health condition, and religion.

Part B: This part has the MAAS, a self-report inventory used to find the level of mindfulness among the undergraduate students of the four faculties. The Mindful Attention Awareness Scale (MAAS) has the longest empirical track record as a valid measure of trait mindfulness (Black et al. 2012). The MAAS has a strongly supported unidimensional factor structure and good nomothetic span (Brown and Ryan 2003; Carlson and Brown 2005; MacKillop and Anderson 2007), making it a seemingly good candidate to represent mindfulness (Van Dam et al. 2010). It has 15 items measuring the degree of awareness of and attention to present moment experience.

Originally, the MAAS comprised a presence and an acceptance factor. The MAAS allows a concise assessment of mindfulness in populations without previous meditation experience. This scale appears to address both the attention and the acceptance aspects of mindfulness, yet does not differentiate one aspect from the other (Bergomi et al. 2013). The MAAS was also found to predict outcomes that are consistent with mindfulness theory (predictive validity) (Michalak et al. 2008). The respondents were expected to rate their experiences based on whether an act performed was done subconsciously or while he/she was preoccupied and not paying attention.

Validity and Reliability of the Instrument

Reliability of an instrument shows its ability to perform and preserve the people or the function of systems in unexpected or repetitive circumstances. Furthermore, it presents the consistency of an instrument for measuring one or some constructs. If the same outcomes have been achieved in applying a test in different conditions or times, then it is a reliable test (Thomas 2009). Reliability aims to demonstrate the trustworthy of the data. A consistent research instrument has every of its item or indicator measuring the same construct; this means that all have been heavily corrected. Factor analyses with undergraduate, community and nationally sampled adult and adult cancer populations have confirmed a single factor scale structure (Brown and Ryan 2003; Carlson and Brown 2005). Previous studies have shown that MAAS has good internal consistency with alphas of more than 0.8 among student and adult samples. The alpha of MAAS in this study during the pilot stage was 0.84.

Validity is the determination of what the researcher wants to measure and how accurate the research results are. In other words, validity is the degree to which the instrument measures what it is supposed to be measuring. Validity indicates the relationship between the test and the behavior that is intended to be measured; it is not defined by a single statistic (Thomas 2009). Again, MAAS has been proven to show good validity in previous studies (Brown and Ryan 2003). The measure takes 5 min or less to complete. A validated, 5-item state version of the MAAS is also available in Brown and Ryan (2003).

3.6 Research Procedure

The defining of objectives is significant in determining what sorts of information are needed to be gathered. This is important in the process of conducting the research to be sure that the results of the study meet the objectives. In this study, once the objectives had been set and that the data needed is determined, related literature and existing resources were reviewed and preliminary tabulation, sampling, and analysis were done to gather data. This step was crucial in nailing the most appropriate survey method which would later govern the validity and reliability of the study outcome (Fig. 3.1).

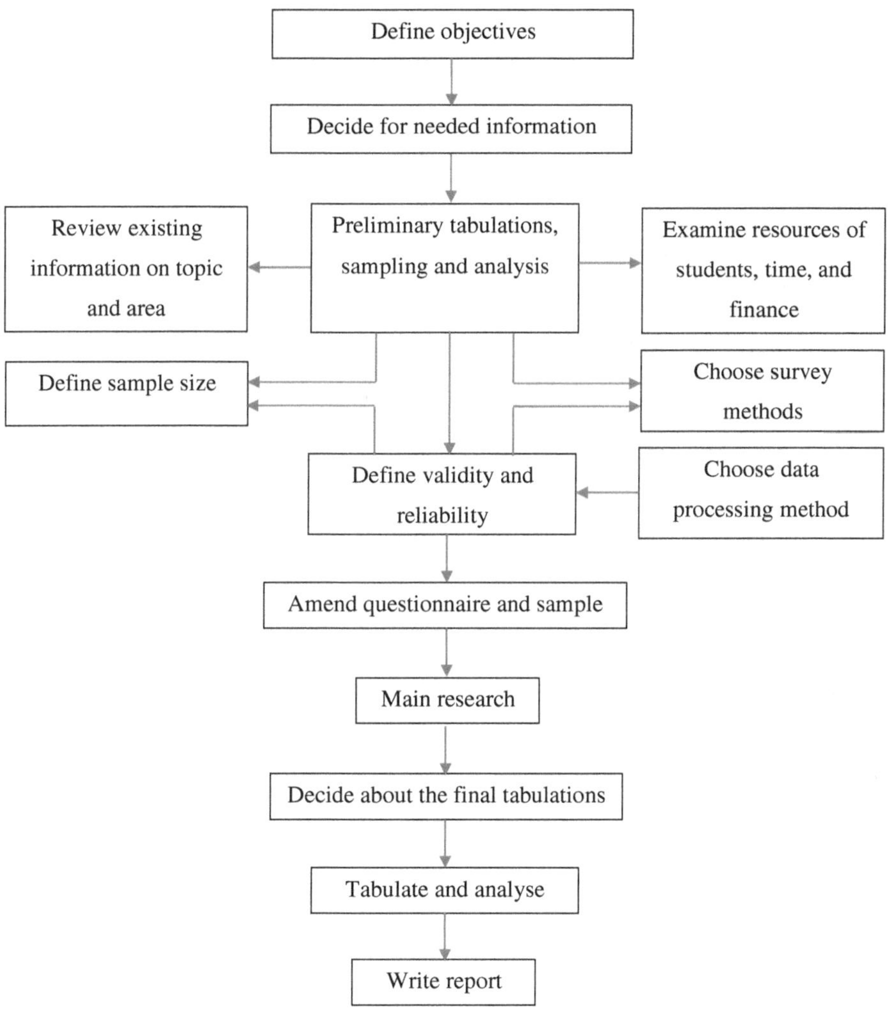

Fig. 3.1 Research procedure

For the purpose of this study, first year undergraduate students in academic year 2012/2013, first semester, were selected. The students were given a brief explanation about the objectives of the study, the aim of the questionnaire, and a quick walk through of the questionnaire. The questionnaire had two parts: Part A asked for the students' demographic information while Part B required the students to answer the MAAS questions.

Rules to maintain good relationship with the respondents were observed during interaction such as giving clear explanation when required and making sure that the environment was comfortable for them to answer the questions.

3.7 Data Process and Analysis

Typically, after data collection, the data are screened (data preparation for analyze), analyzed, and interpreted. This chapter only covers data screening while the other two stages shall be extensively covered in the next chapter. In this research, all data were processed using the Statistical Package for Social Sciences (SPSS) version 19 to facilitate the understanding of data and information gained from the questionnaires. From the point of demographic specifications (gender, age, religion, race, health status, educational back ground, faculty, and family status) and type of faculty (Science, Management, Education, and Civil Engineering), descriptive analyses (percentage and frequency) had been used. Additionally, for clarifying (the level of mindfulness mean, mode, maximum, and minimum was calculated by the software. Correlation analyses illustrated the relationship between demographic factors and type of faculty and the level of mindfulness.

3.8 Conclusion

This chapter discussed the methodology that was utilized for the study execution and explained how this study was conducted to collect reliable data and analyze it to understand the relationship between mindfulness and demographic factors among UTM undergraduate students. In order to meet the objectives of this study, exploratory quantitative method was used because it enabled the researcher to investigate close and new knowledge with economically reasonable cost. Demographic factors and MAAS questionnaires were incorporated into a customized questionnaire to collect the data from 300 undergraduate students of four faculties selected through multiple sampling (Science Faculty, Education Faculty, Management Faculty, and Civil Engineering Faculty). The data were analyzed in descriptive statistics (frequency and percentage) using SPSS 19.

References

Bergomi, C., Tschacher, W., & Kupper, Z. (2013). The assessment of mindfulness with self-report measures: Existing scales and open issues. *Mindfulness, 4*(3), 191–202.

Black, D. S., Sussman, S., Johnson, C. A., & Milam, J. (2012). Psychometric assessment of the mindful attention awareness scale (MAAS) among Chinese adolescents. *Assessment, 19*(1), 42–52.

Brown, K. W., & Ryan, R. M. (2003). The benefits of being present: Mindfulness and its role in psychological well-being. *Journal of Personality and Social Psychology, 84*(4), 822–848.

Carlson, L. E., & Brown, K. W. (2005). Validation of the Mindful Attention Awareness Scale in a cancer population. *Journal of Psychosomatic Research, 58*, 29–33.

Gall, M. D., Gall, J. P., & Borg, W. (2003). *Educational research, an introduction*. Boston: Person Education.

Gay, L. R., Mills, G., & Airasian, P. (2006). *Educational Research. Competencies for analysis and applications* (8th ed.). Pearson.

Grossman, P. (2011). Defining mindfulness by how poorly I think I pay attention during everyday awareness and other intractable problems for psychology's (re)invention of mindfulness: Comment on Brown et al. (2011). *Psychological Assessment, 23*

Grossman, P. (2008). On measuring mindfulness in psychosomatic and psychological research. *Journal of Psychosomatic Research, 64*(4), 405–408.

MacKillop, J., & Anderson, E. J. (2007). Further psychometric validation of the mindful attention awareness scale (MAAS). *Journal of Psychopathology and Behavioral Assessment, 29*(4), 289–293.

Michalak, J., Heidenreich, T., Meibert, P., & Schulte, D. (2008). Mindfulness predicts relapse/recurrence in major depressive disorder following MBCT. *The Journal of Nervous and Mental Disease, 196*, 630–633.

Sekaran, U. (2003). *Research methods for business. A skill building approach* (4th ed.). Wiley.

Thomas, G. (2009). How to do your research project.

Van Dam, N. T., Earleywine, M., & Borders, A. (2010). Measuring mindfulness? An item response theory analysis of the mindful attention awareness scale. *Personality and Individual Differences, 49*(7), 805–810.

Chapter 4
Data Analysis

Abstract Data analysis showed the level of mindfulness among undergraduate students of University technology Malaysia in 2012 is 3.77. In addition, independent variables (age, gender, health condition, family status, educational level, race, religion and type of faculty) only health condition had relationship with the level of mindfulness. Then, first and third null hypothesis were rejected and second one was accepted.

Keywords Results of data analysis · Reject · Accept · Hypothesis

4.1 Introduction

This chapter discusses the data analysis done on the collected data. The achieved results of the questionnaires are described in three main parts—the demography of the respondents, the analysis of mindfulness level, and the analysis results of SPSS, version 19.

4.2 Analysis of Demographic Factors

This section explains the demography of the respondents of the study, which included their gender, age, religion, race, health status, educational back ground, faculty, and family status. This shall be reported in eight tables based on the factors as follows.

4.2.1 Gender

Table 4.1 shows that 73.3 % of the 273 participants of this study were female respondents (n = 200) and 26.7 % were male (n = 73). The higher number of female respondents was not intentional at the time of distribution of the questionnaires.

A. Ahmadi, *Mindfulness Among Students*, SpringerBriefs in Well-Being and Quality of Life Research, DOI 10.1007/978-981-10-2781-9_4

Table 4.1 Number of respondents based on gender

Gender	Frequency	Percentage
Female	200	73.3
Male	73	26.7
Total	273	100

Table 4.2 Number of respondents based on age

Age	Frequency	Percentage (%)
17–21	231	84.6
22–26	33	12.1
27–31	4	1.5
Above	5	1.8
Total	273	100

4.2.2 *Age*

Table 4.2 presents the age of the respondents. In this regard, 84.6 % of 273 participants were 17–21 years old ($n = 231$), 12.1 % were 22–26 years ($n = 33$), 1.5 % were 27–31 years old (n = 4) and 1.8 % were above than 31 years old ($n = 5$). Based on these results, most of the respondents were 17–21 years old.

4.2.3 *Race*

Table 4.3 presents the race composition of the respondents. In this regard, 80.2 % of 273 participants were Malay ($n = 219$), 9.2 % were Chinese ($n = 25$), 1.1 % were Indian and 6.6 % were from other races ($n = 18$). 2.9 % of 273 participants did not answer this question ($n = 8$). The results concluded that most respondents were Malays.

Table 4.3 Number of respondents based on race

Race	Frequency	Percentage (%)
Malay	219	80.2
Chinese	25	9.2
Indian	3	1.1
Else	18	6.6
Total	273	100

Table 4.4 Number of respondents based on religion

Religion	Frequency	Percentage (%)
Islam	238	87.2
Christianity	14	5.1
Buddhism	16	5.9
Hinduism	1	0.4
Irreligion	0	0
Else	3	1.1
Total	273	100

4.2.4 *Religion*

Table 4.4 shows the number of respondents based on religion. 87.2 % of the 273 participants' religion is Islam (n = 238), 5.1 % is Christianity (n = 14), 5.9 % is Buddhism (n = 16), 0.4 % is Hinduism (n = 1), none of the participants' religion is Irreligion (n = 0) and 1.1 % participants are from other religions (n = 3). Based on this table, most of the respondents' religion is Islam.

4.2.5 *Educational Background*

Table 4.5 presents number of respondents based on educational background. 60.4 % of the 273 participants were from Matriculation (n = 165), 15.4 % had a diploma (n = 42), 12.8 % were from STPM/STAM (n = 35) and 10.6 % were from other backgrounds (n = 29). This clearly shows that most students were from Matriculation.

4.2.6 *Types of Faculty*

Table 4.6 depicts the faculties of all 273 respondents where most are first year students from the Faculty of Education (27.5 %, n = 75). Other students were from, in descending order, Faculty of Civil Engineering (27.1 %, n = 74), Faculty of Science (26 %, n = 71), and lastly Faculty of Management (19.4 %, n = 53).

Table 4.5 Number of respondents based on educational background

Educational background	Frequency	Percentage (%)
Matriculation	165	60.4
Diploma	42	15.4
STPM/STAM	35	12.8
Else	29	10.6
Total	273	100

Table 4.6 Number of respondents based on faculty

Faculty	Frequency	Percentage (%)
Science	71	26
Civil Engineering	74	27.1
Management	53	19.4
Education	75	27.5
Total	273	100

Table 4.7 Number of respondents based on family status

Family status	Frequency	Percentage (%)
Both parents	252	92.3
No parents	1	0.4
Single parents	18	6.6
Total	273	100

4.2.7 Family Status

Table 4.7 shows that 92.3 % or $n = 252$ respondents have both parents alive. One student (0.4 %) has no parents while the rest (6.6 %, $n = 18$) only have one parent. The respondents were not required to provide further information on this.

4.2.8 Health Condition

Table 4.8 reveals that 220 respondents (80.6 %) were healthy at the point of study while three of the total 273 respondents (1 %) expressed having physical and psychological problems. 10.3 % had physical problem ($n = 28$) and 7 % reported psychological problem ($n = 19$).

4.2.9 Relationship Between Mindfulness Level and Demographic Factors

Table 4.9 shows the overall relationship between mindfulness level and gender, age, race, educational background, religion, and family condition. No significant relationship has been detected.

Table 4.8 Number of respondents based on health condition

Health condition	Frequency	Percentage (%)
Physical problem	28	10.3
Psychological problem	19	7
None of above	220	80.6
Both	3	1
Total	273	100

Table 4.9 Relationship between mindfulness level and demographic factors (except health)

		MFMean
MFMean	Pearson Correlation	1
	Sig. (2-tailed) N	273
Gender	Pearson Correlation	0.053
	Sig. (2-tailed) N	0.379273
Age	Pearson Correlation	−0.048
	Sig. (2-tailed) N	0.427273
Religion	Pearson Correlation	0.054
	Sig. (2-tailed) N	0.370273
Race	Pearson correlation	−0.020
	Sig. (2-tailed) N	0.742273
Education	Pearson correlation	0.026
	Sig. (2-tailed) N	0.671273
Family	Pearson correlation	−0.057
	Sig. (2-tailed) N	0.345273

Table 4.10 Relationship between mindfulness level and health condition

		MFMean	Health
Spearman's rho	Correlation	1.000	0.124*
	Coefficient Sig. (2-tailed) N	0.273	0.040273
	Correlation	0.124*	1.000
	Coefficient Sig. (2-tailed) N	0.040273	0.273

*correlation is significant at the 0.05 level (2-tailed)

Table 4.10 highlights that the relationship between mindfulness level and health condition is not significant.

4.3 Level of Mindfulness Based on Individual

Table 4.11 summarizes the mean, mode, maximum, and minimum scores of the 273 respondents in terms of their mindfulness level according to the MAAS questionnaire. On average, the students scored 3.77 on the scale and most scored 3.73. The maximum score was 5.87 while the lowest score was 1.

Table 4.11 Level of mindfulness of the respondents

Mean of mindfulness scores in the sample	3.77
Mode of mindfulness scores in the sample	3.73
Maximum mindfulness scores in the sample	5.87
Minimum mindfulness scores in the sample	1

Table 4.12 Level of mindfulness based on faculty

Faculty	Mean	*n*	Std. deviation
Science	3.8218	71	0.66
Management	3.6347	53	0.64
Education	3.8203	75	0.73
Civil engineering	3.7747	74	0.73
Total	3.7723	273	0.70

Table 4.13 Relationship between level of mindfulness and type of faculty

		MFMean	Faculty
MFMean	Pearson correlation	1	0.002
	Sig. (2-tailed) N	273	0.973273
Faculty	Pearson correlation	0.002	1
	Sig. (2-tailed) N	0.973273	273

4.4 Level of Mindfulness Based on Faculty

On average, students from the Faculty of Science scored the highest in level of mindfulness (3.82) based on the results depicted in Table 4.12. In the Management Faculty, this was 3.6347 ($n = 53$), in the Education Faculty was 3.8203 ($n = 75$) and in the Civil Engineering Faculty was 3.77 ($n = 74$). Students from the Management Faculty scored the lowest.

4.4.1 Relationship Between Level of Mindfulness and Type of Faculty

Table 4.13 shows that there is no relationship between the level of mindfulness and type of faculty.

4.5 Analysis of Hypotheses

The three hypotheses tested in this study were null hypotheses, which were hypotheses that offered no statistical significant difference in a set of proposed conditions. This was to show that no variation between variables existed, and was expected to be true until statistical evidence would reject it for an alternative hypothesis.

4.5.1 First Hypothesis

First null hypothesis: The level of mindfulness among UTM first year undergraduate students is the same as the general population.

This null hypothesis was rejected because the level of mindfulness in undergraduate students was 3.77, which was less than that of the general population (3.86). Therefore, the alternative hypothesis which states otherwise, i.e., the level of mindfulness among UTM first year undergraduate students is not the same as the general population was accepted.

4.5.2 Second Hypothesis

Second null hypothesis: There is no relationship between type of faculty and the level of mindfulness among first year undergraduate students of UTM.

This hypothesis was accepted because there was no any significant relationship between type of faculty and the level of mindfulness.

4.5.3 Third Hypothesis

Third null hypothesis: There is no relationship between the level of mindfulness and demographic factors among first year undergraduate students of UTM.

The null hypothesis was not rejected fully in this sense based on the following results obtained from data analysis:

1. There was no relationship between age and the level of mindfulness.
2. There was no relationship between gender and the level of mindfulness.
3. There was no relationship between educational background and the level of mindfulness.
4. There was no relationship between family status and the level of mindfulness.
5. There was no relationship between religion and the level of mindfulness.
6. There was a relationship between health condition and the level of mindfulness.
7. There was no relationship between race and the level of mindfulness.

4.6 Conclusion

The data analysis results showed that not all null hypotheses have been accepted; one null hypothesis was rejected, one was accepted, and the last one was partially accepted. These conclusions were reached after analyzing all data as per detailed out in Chap. 3 and then tabulating the results as per Tables 4.1, 4.2, 4.3, 4.4, 4.5, 4.6, 4.7, 4.8, 4.9, 4.10, 4.11, 4.12 and 4.13. Nevertheless, the objectives of this study had been achieved, which were to: (1) identify the level of mindfulness among first year undergraduate students of UTM in 2012; (2) identify the relationship between type of faculty and the level of mindfulness among first year undergraduate students of UTM; and (3) identify the relationship between demographic factors and the level of mindfulness among first year undergraduate students of UTM. The next chapter shall put forth more detailed interpretation of the analyzed data, supported by an in-dept discussion. The results of this study can be used as a guideline for psychologists, counselors, medical doctors, responsible of university, health ministries and other researchers for more similar investigations.

Chapter 5
Discussion, Implication, and Conclusion

Abstract This chapter discussed organizational environment, entrance into a new challenging organization and physical and psychological status could lead to low level of mindfulness among the participants. Interestingly, subject of study besides different type of contents, had lower impact than individual characteristics on the mindfulness. Implications of the study for universities, students and researcher were stated. Recommandations for governmental policies, body of knowledge, and theory developing as well as work of practitionnaires was in parallel with discussed issues.

Keywords Discussion · Recommendation · Implication · Limitation

5.1 Introduction

This chapter is put forth to answer the research questions posed earlier based on the data analysis results previously shown in Chap. 4 and in accordance to published theories and its literature. To recap, these research questions were:

1. What is the level of mindfulness among UTM first year undergraduate students?
2. What is the relationship between the level of mindfulness among UTM first year undergraduate students and type of faculty?
3. What is the relationship between the level of mindfulness and demographic factors among UTM first year undergraduate students? The factors investigated were gender, age, religion, race, educational background, health condition, and family status.

It should be emphasized here that all data was quantitatively collected using a customized questionnaire asking for the respondent's demographic information and also their responses to the MAAS questionnaire developed by Brown and Ryan (2003). The sample of this study was 273 first year undergraduate students from

A. Ahmadi, *Mindfulness Among Students*, SpringerBriefs in Well-Being and Quality of Life Research, DOI 10.1007/978-981-10-2781-9_5

four different faculties who, at the point of this study, were in their first semester in UTM. As such, all discussions hereafter shall be focused on their responses in the aforementioned customized questionnaire and its analysis results from SPSS version 19.

5.2 Level of Mindfulness Among UTM Undergraduate Students

Mindfulness is an inherent human capacity that occurs naturally (Brown and Ryan 2004; Goldstein 2002; Kabat-Zinn 2003) and developed by a combination of concentrative and analytical insight-based skills. It entails the ability to flexibly apportion between primary attention to the foreground and secondary awareness to the background (Rapgay and Bystrisky 2009; Teasdale et al. 2002; Van Dam et al. 2010). This study had discovered that the level of mindfulness among the undergraduate students was 3.77, which was less than that of the general population (3.86). This finding can be generalized to the undergraduate students from other universities as well on the basis that, as mentioned by some studies, the students were still adapting to the new university environment, which also affected their minds. The new environment brings forth new people, social status, and an education structure completely different from their high schools. So, it is the natural defence of mind to change the power of attention and awareness, and only the more mindful students are able to maintain their abilities of maintaining mental stability.

Obvious changes in the entity of life can induce challenges. Entering university (as a higher level of education) can adversely affect one's academic achievement due to a disturbed mind (Beauchemin et al. 2008), and the effect is more profound among undergraduate students who suddenly find a steep change in their learning environment (Feldman et al. 2007). Undergraduate students in the first semester can be one of high risk groups whose mindfulness level can be disturbed besides being exposed, or already exposed, to other mental difficulties (Lynch et al. 2011).

By guiding people to accept thoughts and feelings without judgment and to focus on the present moment, cognitive reappraisal ability will improve (Troy et al. 2013). To increase the level of mindfulness, mindfulness mediation and self-regulation practices are recommended. These are also helpful to undergraduate students. Other suggested practices include practicing attention and awareness to bring mental processes under self-control, fostering mental well-being, and developing specific capacities (such as calmness, clarity and concentration) (Walsh and Shapiro 2006). This is in view that mindfulness is not only positively correlated with empathy, but also self-awareness (Beitel et al. 2005). Additional factors related to higher level of mindfulness are emotional intelligence, attention to feelings and clarity of feelings. This means that mood repair, attention to emotions, and openness to experience are helpful to develop mindfulness as well. Life satisfaction and conscientiousness can improve awareness of human (Baer 2015; Baer et al. 2004; Brown and Ryan 2003).

The lowest level of mindfulness among the respondents was 1 (The minimum level that can be achieved by this inventory is also 1). The first possible reason for this is that the respondents have given careless answers which do not portray their true potential. This is because, for an emerging adult who has been accepted into a university, such score is impossible since the student cannot be illiterate. Otherwise, it may mean that the students were suffering from severe psychological diseases that have disrupted their attention, awareness, and judgment; such patients can hardly live a normal life to begin with. The conditions here may refer to brain injury (Hart et al. 2005), severe anxiety, severe depression, bipolar disorders, schizophrenia, addictions, ADHD (Sadock et al. 2007) and dyslexia.

The highest level of mindfulness was 5.87 (The maximum level that can be achieved by this inventory is 6). The students who have achieved such high level of mindfulness are perceived as having powerful psychological abilities in preserving attention and awareness as well as making sound judgment. In addition, they have considerable self-control since mindfulness increases psychological well-being by reducing general distress after accounting for self-control. In other words, mindfulness is a moderator of the correlation between self-control and psychological symptoms (Bowlin and Baer 2012).

Increasing mindfulness is a prominent issue in today's world. It is a necessity for proper achievement in not only vocation, but also in daily common life's goals. Mindfulness is a key component of being human as it involves consciousness and awareness. It is fundamentally about cultivating awareness and attention, and has significant relevance to personal quality of life and well-being (Ludwig and Kabat-Zinn 2008; Ruff and Elizabeth 2009).

5.3 The Relationship Between Level of Mindfulness and Type of Faculty

The analysis results had shown no significant relationship between level of mindfulness and type of faculty. This result is supported by few previous studies investigate the relationship between field of study and response to mindfulness-training programs (Shapiro et al. 1998). This is attributed to the fact that the process of teaching and learning in all faculties of UTM is the same, which means there is no difference between challenges and issues that students confront other than a difference in the course content. So, the influence of type of faculty in the level of mindfulness is insignificant. In addition, undergraduate students in their first semester do not face significant or specified subjects that can induce changes in their attention and awareness status. Nevertheless, such low level of awareness in all four scrutinized faculties is a worrying phenomenon which can mean that the teaching and learning strategies in UTM are not effective enough to stimulate the organizational part of their mindfulness.

The lowest level of mindfulness among the faculties was 3.63 in the Faculty of Management. This may be caused by the mindless programs, disciplines and policies embedded in their course. The curriculums can influence their organizational mindfulness because interesting context is able to improve foresight and mind power. Continuous scrutiny towards thoughts and beliefs; refinement of expectations based on the moment experiences; and appreciation of the subtleties of the events are positive consequences of mindful minds (Hoy and Tschannen-Moran 2007; Langer and Piper 1987). Attributes which demonstrate mindfulness and are encouraged to be embedded in the course include being prepared for defeat, sensitive to quality, reluctant to simplify, being resilient, and able to greaten the expertise (Weick and Sutcliffe 2001). Not only that, as mentioned by Bowlin and Baer (2012), organizational mindfulness results in better self-control to promote mental wellbeing through distress reduction (Crane et al. 2010; Williams et al. 2011).

The highest level of mindfulness among the faculties was 3.82 in the Faculty of Science. It seems that the students of this faculty have higher psychological abilities in paying attention, being awareness, and making judgement. This may be related to the subjects offered in the faculty which demand the students to be innovative and practical.

Mindfulness requires vigilance, flexibility, and the ability to break set. So the strict principles of the faculties may limit the level of mindfulness; this has been supported by some studies which mentioned that education could abound in mindlessness by rigid bureaucracies (Langer and Moldoveanu 2000) and mindless standardization (Hoy and Tschannen-Moran 2007). Relying on standard practices and routines protect organizational functioning from the vagaries and novelty, but good organizational environments could promote thoughtful adaptability and cultivate mindful actions.

To enhance mindfulness, students need to feel free to experiment and not be afraid of making mistakes. They must have the confidence and be encouraged to take risks and break new grounds. Every university and faculty administrator should understand the importance of mindfulness for mental hygiene of students, practise it, and lead students in mindful ways. With better mental health, students' academic achievement can become better and this will ultimately benefit the university. The students will also bring forth positive energy and create a happy atmosphere in the faculty. Participating in programs that increase mindfulness could improve their quality of life (Crane and Kuyken 2013; Raes et al. 2014).

5.4 The Relationship Between Level of Mindfulness and Demographic Factors

Mindfulness cannot be taught in academic settings because it is a personal, internal, dynamic, and experiential process. Thus, demographic factors can be related to the lack or low level of mindfulness because these kinds of human characteristics may affect the mind. However, this study has found no significant relationship between level of mindfulness and most demographic factors except a positive relationship with health condition among the 273 UTM students.

The finding of this study contradicts with some previous studies. For instance, gender has been found to influence mindfulness. In the study by Marison, women showed lower mindfulness level than men. Difference in sexual steroid concentration (particularly estrogens), has also been found to contribute to the gender difference in adaptability and stress responsiveness (Pico-Alfonso et al. 2007). On the other hand, in the study of Soysa and Wilcomb (2015) undergraduate self-reports of the four facets of mindfulness (describing, awareness, non-judging, and non reactivity) did not vary by gender. When the facets of mindfulness were added in their study, were not predicted by gender.

In terms of age, some studies have found lower mindfulness level among older people. Baer (2008) opined that the effect is caused by the mind's ability to judge and concentrate, which is often better among younger people. Although Dundas et al. (2013) found that older students achieved higher scores of MAAS and FFMQ. Again, this has not shown much difference in this study because the respondents' age range is narrow. Also, everyone has the same educational status at the point of study, which may the reason that they have spent equal time and concentration in answering the questionnaire.

Religion is a set of belief and cultural systems. It is a world view including established symbols that relates humanity to moral values and spirituality. The worship of and the belief in the power of a controlling superhuman, especially a God, can establish mind abilities (Hill 1973). In regard to religion, this is the first study which has critically investigated the relationship between mindfulness and many religions. Previous studies mostly stated the importance of mindfulness in each religion and its influence in some religions only. In this study, the effect of culture on the people's attitude towards religion and mind abilities are more dominant that the religion's influence on the people's level of mindfulness. Thus, a relationship between religion and the level of mindfulness was not significant.

Similar to the effect of gender, race seems to be influencing the level of mindfulness in some reported works, but again, this study has found no correlation between these two variables. Similarly, in the study of Cresswell et al. (2007), dispositional mindfulness was not associated with ethnicity when comparison was made between Asians and other ethnic groups. The possible reason may be that the Malaysian society is integrated and has formed a unique 'Malaysian culture'. In other studies, the different races may not integrate to that extent.

Educational level was not significantly associated with the scores from MAAS (Schmertz 2008). Though relationship has yet to be extensively studied in most published works, some have pointed out the following: *Education levels did not differ significantly between the meditators of mindfulness training and non-mediators* (Lykins and Baer 2009). Also, the impact of mindfulness training on academic performance, self-concept and anxiety was found to be positive (Franco et al. 2010).

A positive correlation between perceived health and mindfulness and also between psychological well-being and mindfulness was found in this study. The reason is obvious where compromised health condition affects one's attention and awareness. Positive psychological effects of mindfulness include reductions in a variety of problematic conditions (Baer 2003; Grossman et al. 2004) and improved cognition (Zeidan et al. 2010), better subjective well-being and improved behavioral regulation as well as reduced emotional reactivity and psychological symptoms (Keng et al. 2011). High mindfulness on the MAAS was shown to correlate positively with self-rated health in some other studies (Dundas et al. 2013).

Traditional dualistic views of the mind-body among health practitioners and their underlying connection are slowly being accepted. More are interested in knowing how mindfulness, as a form of consciousness naturally develops, can flourish in despite of individual differences in propensity and willingness to be mindful (Brown and Ryan 2003). Mindfulness helps a person to accept existing conditions in action, even the act of self-criticizing as a way towards self-acceptance (Germer et al. 2005). Some training, particularly meditation, have been proven to improve mindfulness (Davidson et al. 2003; Shapiro et al. 2008). Being happy, healthy, and satisfied in the present life promotes the level of mindfulness. Becoming kind, keeping thoughtful relationships, and having small amount of possessions are the consequence of a mindful life.

5.5 Implications

The findings of this study are useful for universities, body of knowledge, counselors, psychologists and psychiatrists. Since undergraduate students form the major community in universities, the results can bring a good insight into their level of mindfulness. This study has contributed a new literature to the relationship between demographic factors and level of mindfulness through a quantitative survey. In addition, it seems that this is the first attempt in examining the relationship between the level of mindfulness and type of faculty.

This study has found a positive relationship between mindfulness level and health condition. Mindfulness as a psychological function can ameliorate a variety of conditions such as personality disorders, anxiety, substance abuse, stress, as well as chronic pain and adaptive coping (Burke 2010; Chiesa and Serretti 2011;

Fjorback et al. 2011; Halland et al. 2015; Hofmann et al. 2010; Mars and Abbey 2010; Sauer et al. 2013; Walach et al. 2012). This means that a student's health, both mentally and physically, plays a crucial part in helping them to cope with their new environment once they enter university. Promoting the faculty's curriculums and interactions of administrations with students together with creating novelty in programs could increase organizational mindfulness of the new students. Mindfulness serves as a strong tool in teaching, learning, and leadership processes within higher education settings (Davis 2014).

Providing empathically acknowledging experience, taking action toward change and decision making, teaching students how to respond rather than react to the core issues in their lives, establishing personal boundaries; developing environmental awareness; providing healthful nutrition and facilities for caring of the body; recognizing inner strengths; restoring life balance through rest, relaxation, and recreation; building supportive relationships; and discovering passions and envisioning goals are positive roles of universities for their students to improve their level of mindfulness (Napoli and Bonifas 2011; Napoli 2010; Napoli and Roe 2008).

Wellbeing, on the other hand, includes the physical, social and emotional dimensions of a person's state. A healthy wellbeing implies that the basic needs of individuals are met, that they have a sense of purpose and are able to achieve important personal goals and socialise in the society. A healthier and productive environment in the campus, including the need to have enough counselors, psychologists, social workers and trainers to assist in the undergraduate students' mental health and wellbeing must be put in place in the university. Stress and anger management training, healthier lifestyles training, emotional resilience training, and mentoring programmes ought to be available to help the students develop a healthy resilient lifestyle (Mey and Yin 2015).

5.6 Recommendations

The recommendations put forth her have been generalized according to the major findings and related theories to promote the level of mindfulness among undergraduate students and factors that are related to the level of mindfulness. Theory development, the government policies, and the work of practitioners are three main parts of recommendation in this chapter. Fundamentally, improvement of the level of mindfulness and providing additional literature in this research area among undergraduate students are recommended. Promoting good and healthy habits are also encouraged to improve the students' mental health. The results of this study have also emphasized that a student's mental health cannot be solely judged based on his or her demographic characteristics.

5.6.1 Recommendation for the Government Policies

Students are recommended to keep track of their own mental and physical health before joining the university. They are also encouraged to join activities which promote mindfulness and other psychologically similar programs. With this, more replication of similar studies can be made and be expanded to include postgraduate students and more international students to understand their level of mindfulness. Moreover, it makes the identification of other factors which affect mindfulness level possible to further enhance university students' mental and physical health.

In order to improve the academic achievement and organizational mindfulness in the faculties, the administration is recommended to hold mindfulness training programs, seminars, and workshops (Palmer and Rodger 2009). A shift of mindset from old mindless educational system to more mindful system is also encouraged. Also, providing more places of entertainment and relaxation for students in the faculties can be useful in reducing stress.

In order to establish a mindful university as a successful higher educational institution, it is recommended to deepen the existing information regarding the students' mental health. University Counseling Centers are important places to hold educational and training programs to increase the knowledge of students about their physical and mental health problems. Being mindful and mindfulness practices (sitting meditation, walking meditation, yoga, and qigong), can promote mental health and physical well-being (Englund-Helmeke 2014; Farb et al. 2007; Tang et al. 2007). A program with formal meditations and informal practice may be a more promising intervention for university student stress than one with brief mindfulness exercises and informal practice (Hindman et al. 2015).

5.6.2 Recommendation for the Work of Practitioners

Mindfulness relates to coping styles, thereby it is recommended to counselors, general physicians, psychiatrists, and psychologists to pay attention to the high risk groups with low mindfulness (first year students during often difficult transition to university) who may have other problems and issues leading to the low mindfulness or vice versa. Interventions led to increases in mindfulness, primarily decrease rumination and increased emotional clarity (Caldwell and Shaver 2015). Application of instruments (such as MASS as a reliable and valid inventory) helps to illustrate the level of mindfulness among their patients and clients. The process of self-monitoring and self-reporting of mindfulness alone can produce desirable behavior change (Bergomi et al. 2013; Korotitsch and Nelson-Gray 1999). To enhance the level of mindfulness, health condition should be improved. Furthermore, mindfulness training programs, related seminars and workshop are beneficial.

5.6.3 *Recommendation for Body of Knowledge and Theory Development*

It is recommended to the body of knowledge to add more literature on mindfulness and its predictors through quantitative and qualitative methods and to add literature on the level of mindfulness across group (Walker 2011), differentiate it with other variables relevant for health and well-beingtrace (Koenig 2008) and embrace novel facets of mindfulness (Griffiths et al. 2009) and related factors.

5.7 Limitation of the Study

Application of qualitative and quantitative method provides more accurate information for identifying the level of mindfulness and related factor. The study was among four faculties in UTM. Hence, it is recommended that more faculties in different universities be included in similar studies.

5.8 Conclusion

This chapter has interpreted and discussed the findings of this study based on the objectives of the study, which are to identify the level of mindfulness among first year undergraduate students and its relationship with some demographic factors. Comparison and reference have been made to some published works. The level of mindfulness among undergraduate students of UTM was less than the general population, and the only related demographic factor to this level was the students' health condition. Type of faculty, regardless of whether it is a Science or Arts faculty, was not correlated to the level of mindfulness. The implications of the study were briefly stated and relevant recommendations were given thereafter. The limitation of this study as previously stated should not be ignored and suggestions have been given to improve future studies.

Mindfulness continues to gain empirical support as an important construct in the field of mental health. Because this study used quantitative method and used the MAAS among the university students, research can progress to examine the empirical relationships between mindfulness and other factors including mental and behavioral health among this population. The current study provided initial evidence that the MAAS was positively correlated with health and suggests that trait mindfulness has a promising future for etiological studies among different populations. Future research should use methods to determine if the MAAS remains sound measures among other populations.

References

Baer, R. (2003). Mindfulness training as a clinical intervention: A conceptual and empirical review. *Clinical Psychology: Science and Practice, 10*, 125–143.

Baer, R. (2008). Construct validity of the five facet mindfulness questionnaire in meditating and none meditating samples. *Assessment, 15*(3), 329–342.

Baer, R. A. (Ed.). (2015). *Mindfulness-based treatment approaches: Clinician's guide to evidence base and applications*. United States: Academic Press.

Baer, R., Smith, G., & Allen, K. (2004). Assessment of mindfulness by self-report The Kentucky inventory of mindfulness skills. *Assess, 11*, 191–206.

Beauchemin, J., Hutchins, T. L., & Patterson, F. (2008). Mindfulness meditation may lessen anxiety, promote social skills, and improve academic performance among adolescents with learning disabilities. *Journal of Evidence Based Complementary and Alternative Medicine, 13*(1), 34–45.

Beitel, M., Ferrer, E., & Cecero, J. J. (2005). Psychological mindedness and awareness of self and others. *Journal of Clinical Psychology, 61*(6), 739–750.

Bergomi, C., Tschacher, W., & Kupper, Z. (2013). The assessment of mindfulness with self-report measures: Existing scales and open issues. *Mindfulness, 4*(3), 191–202.

Bowlin, S. L., & Baer, R. A. (2012). Relationships between mindfulness, self-control, and psychological functioning. *Personality and Individual Differences, 52*(3), 411–415.

Brown, K. W., & Ryan, R. M. (2003). The benefits of being present: Mindfulness and its role in psychological well-being. *Journal of Personality and Social Psychology, 84*(4), 822–848.

Brown, K. W., & Ryan, R. M. (2004). Perils and promises in defining and measuring mindfulness: Observations from experience. *Clinical Psychology: Science and Practice, 11*, 242–248.

Burke, C. A. (2010). Mindfulness-based approaches with children and adolescents: A preliminary review of current research in an emergent field. *Journal of Child and Family Studies, 19*(2), 133–144.

Caldwell, J. G., & Shaver, P. R. (2015). Promoting attachment-related mindfulness and compassion: A wait-list-controlled study of women who were mistreated during childhood. *Mindfulness, 6*(3), 624–636.

Chiesa, A., & Serretti, A. (2011). Mindfulness based cognitive therapy for psychiatric disorders: A systematic review and meta-analysis. *Psychiatry Research, 187*(3), 441–453.

Crane, C., Barnhofer, T., Hargus, E., Winder, R., & Amarasinghe, M. (2010). The relationship between mindfulness and conditional goal setting in depressed patients. *British Journal of Clinical Psychology, 42*, 281–290.

Crane, R. S., & Kuyken, W. (2013). The implementation of mindfulness-based cognitive therapy: Learning from the UK health service experience. *Mindfulness, 4*(3), 246–254.

Cresswell, D., David, C., Baldwin, M., Naomi, I., & Matthio, D. (2007). Neural correlates of dispositional mindfulness during affect labeling. *Psychosomatic Medicine, 69*, 560.

Davidson, R. J., Kabat-Zinn, J., Schumacher, J., Rosenkranz, M., Muller, D., Santorelli, S. F. … Sheridan, J. F. (2003). Alterations in brain and immune function produced by mindfulness meditation. *Psychosomatic medicine, 65*(4), 564–570.

Davis, D. J. (2014). Mindfulness in higher education: Teaching, learning, and leadership. *International Journal of Religion and Spirituality in Society*, 4(3).

Dundas, I., Vøllestad, J., Binder, P. E., & Sivertsen, B. (2013). The five factor mindfulness questionnaire in Norway. *Scandinavian Journal of Psychology, 54*(3), 250–260.

Englund-Helmeke., Shawn R. (2014). Mindfulness and Well-Being. *Master of social work clinical research papers*. Paper 313. http://sophia.stkate.edu/msw_papers/313

Farb, N. A., Segal, Z. V., Mayberg, H., Bean, J., McKeon, D., Fatima, Z., et al. (2007). Attending to the present: Mindfulness meditation reveals distinct neural modes of self-reference. *Social Cognitive and Affective Neuroscience, 2*(4), 313–322.

Feldman, G., Hayes, A., Kumar, S., Greeson, J., & Laurenceau, J. (2007). Mindfulness and emotion regulation: The development and initial validation of the cognitive and affective mindfulness scale-revised (CAMS-R). *Journal of Behavioral Assessment, 29*, 177–190.

Fjorback, L., Ørnbøl, E., Rehfeld, E., Arendt, M., Fink, P., & Schröder, A. (2011). Mindfulness therapy for bodily distress syndrome—A randomized controlled trial. *Journal of Psychosomatic Research.*

Franco, C., Mañas, I., Cangas, A., & Gallego, J. (2010). The applications of mindfulness with students of secondary school: Results on the academic performance. *Self-concept and Anxiety, 1*(3), 83–97.

Germer, C. K., Siegel, R., & Fulton, P. (2005). *Mindfulness and psychotherapy*. New York: Guilford Press.

Goldstein, J. (2002). *One dharma: The emerging western Buddhism*. New York: Harper San Francisco.

Griffiths, K., Camic, P. M., & Hutton, J. M. (2009). Participant experiences of a mindfulness-based cognitive therapy group for cardiac rehabilitation. *Journal of Health Psychology, 14*(5), 675–681. doi:10.1177/1359105309104911

Grossman, P., Neimann, L., Schmidt, S., & Walach, H. (2004). Mindfulness-based stress reduction and health benefits: A meta-analysis. *Psychosomatic Research, 57*, 35–43.

Halland, E., de Vibe, M., Solhaug, I., Friborg, O., Rosenvinge, J. H., Tyssen, R. … Bjørndal, A. (2015). Mindfulness training improves problem-focused coping in psychology and medical students: results from a randomized controlled trial. *College Student Journal, 49*(3), 387–398.

Hart, T., Whyte, J., Kim, J., & Vaccaro, M. (2005). Executive function and self-awareness of "real-world" behavior and attention deficits following traumatic brain injury. *The Journal of Head Trauma Rehabilitation, 20*(4), 333–347.

Hill, S. S. (1973). Sociology of religion. *Journal of the American Academy of Religion, 41*(3), 447–450.

Hindman, R. K., Glass, C. R., Arnkoff, D. B., & Maron, D. D. (2015). A comparison of formal and informal mindfulness programs for stress reduction in university students. *Mindfulness, 6*(4), 873–884.

Hofmann, S. G., Sawyer, A. T., Witt, A. A., & Oh, D. (2010). The effect of mindfulness-based therapy on anxiety and depression: A meta analytic review. *Journal of Consulting and Clinical Psychology, 78*(2), 169–183.

Hoy, W. K., & Tschannen-Moran, M. (2007). The conceptualization and measurement of faculty trust in schools. *Essential ideas for the reform of American schools*, 87–114.

Kabat-Zinn, J. (2003). Mindfulness-based interventions in context: Past, present, and future. *Clinical Psychology: Science and Practice, 10*, 144–156.

Keng, S., Smoski, M. J., & Robins, C. J. (2011). Effects of mindfulness on psychological health: A review of empirical studies. *Clinical Psychology: Science and Practice*. doi:10.1016/j.cpr.2011.04.006

Koenig, H. G. (2008). Concerns about measuring "spirituality" in research. *The Journal of Nervous and Mental Disease, 196*(5), 349–355. doi:10.1097/NMD.1090b1013e31816ff31796

Korotitsch, W. J., & Nelson-Gray, R. O. (1999). An overview of self monitoring research in assessment and treatment. *Psychological Assessment, 11*, 415–425.

Langer, E. J., & Moldoveanu, M. (2000). The construct of mindfulness. *Journal of Social Issues, 56*(1), 1–9.

Langer, E. J., & Piper, A. I. (1987). The prevention of mindlessness. *Personality and Social Psychology, 53*, 280–287.

Ludwig, D. S., & Kabat-Zinn, J. (2008). Mindfulness in medicine. *American Medical Association, 300*(11), 1350–1352.

Lykins, E. L., & Baer, R. A. (2009). Psychological functioning in a sample of long-term practitioners of mindfulness meditation. *Journal of Cognitive Psychotherapy, 23*(3), 226–241.

Lynch, S., Gander, M. L., Kohls, N., Kudielka, B., & Walach, H. (2011). Mindfulness based coping with university life: A non-randomized wait-list-controlled pilot evaluation. *Stress and Health, 27*(5), 365–375.

Mars, T. S., & Abbey, H. (2010). Mindfulness meditation practise as a healthcare intervention: A systematic review. *International Journal of Osteopathic Medicine, 13*(2), 56–66.
Mey, S. C., & Yin, C. J. (2015). Mental health and wellbeing of the undergraduate students in a research university: a malaysian experience. *Social Indicators Research, 122*(2), 539–551.
Napoli, M. (2010). *Tools for mindful living: Steppingstones for practice*. Dubuque, IA: Kendall/Hunt Publishing.
Napoli, M., & Bonifas, R. P. (2011). From theory toward empathic self care: Creating a mindful classroom for social work students. *Social Work Education: An International Journal, 30*, 635–649.
Napoli, M., & Roe, S. (2008). *Life by personal design: Limitless horizons*. Dubuque, IA: Kendall/Hunt Publishing.
Palmer, A., & Rodger, S. (2009). Mindfulness, stress, and coping among university students. *Canadian Journal of Counselling, 43*(3), 198.
Pico-Alfonso, A., Mastorci, F., Ceresini, G., Ceda, M., Ghi, M., Pino, O., et al. (2007). Acute psychosocial challenge and cardiac autonomic response in women: The role of estrogens, corticosteroids, and behavioral coping styles. *Psychoneuroendocrinology, 32*, 451–463.
Raes, F., Griffith, J. W., Van der Gucht, K., & Williams, J. M. G. (2014). School-based prevention and reduction of depression in adolescents: A cluster-randomized controlled trial of a mindfulness group program. *Mindfulness, 5*(5), 477–486.
Rapgay, L., & Bystrisky, A. (2009). Classical mindfulness: An introduction to its theory and practice for clinical application. *Annals of the New York Academy of Sciences, 1172*, 148–162.
Ruff, M., & Elizabeth, R. (2009). The role of mindfulness in healthcare reform: A policy paper. 313–323 (Mackenzie, Guest Editorial).
Sadock, B. J., Sadock, V. A., & Levin, Z. E. (Eds.). (2007). *Kaplan and Sadock's study guide and self-examination review in psychiatry*. Philadelphia: Lippincott Williams & Wilkins.
Sauer, S. et al. (2013). Assessment of mindfulness: Review on state of the art. *Mindfulness, 4*(1), 3–17.
Schmertz, S. (2008). Rumination as a mediator of the relation between mindfulness and social anxiety in a clinical sample. Dissertation. Georgia State University.
Shapiro, S., Oman, D., Thoresen, C., Plante, T., & Flinders, T. (2008). Cultivating mindfulness: Effects on well-being. *Clinical Psychology: Science and Practice, 64*(840–862), 67.
Shapiro, S. L., Schwartz, G. E., & Bonner, G. (1998). Effects of mindfulness-based stress reduction on medical and premedical students. *Journal of Behavioral Medicine, 21*(6), 581–599.
Soysa, C. K., & Wilcomb, C. J. (2015). Mindfulness, self-compassion, self-efficacy, and gender as predictors of depression, anxiety, stress, and well-being. *Mindfulness, 6*(2), 217–226.
Tang, Y. Y., Ma, Y., Wang, J., Fan, Y., Feng, S., Lu, Q. … Posner, M. I. (2007). Short-term meditation training improves attention and self-regulation. *Proceedings of the National Academy of Sciences, 104*(43), 17152–17156.
Teasdale, J. D., Moore, R. G., Hayhurst, H., Pope, M., Williams, S., & Segal, Z. V. (2002). Metacognitive awareness and prevention of relapse in depression: Empirical evidence. *Journal of Consulting and Clinical Psychology, 70*, 275–287.
Troy, A. S., Shallcross, A. J., Davis, T. S., & Mauss, I. B. (2013). History of mindfulness-based cognitive therapy is associated with increased cognitive reappraisal ability. *Mindfulness, 4*(3), 213–222.
Van Dam, N. T., Earleywine, M., & Borders, A. (2010). Measuring mindfulness? An item response theory analysis of the mindful attention awareness scale. *Personality and Individual Differences, 49*(7), 805–810.
Walach, H., Ferrari, M. L. G., Sauer, S., & Kohls, N. (2012). Mind-body practices in integrative medicine. *Religions, 3*(1), 50–81.
Walker, C. M. (2011). What's the DIF? Why differential item functioning analyses are an important part of instrument development and validation. *Journal of Psychoeducational Assessment, 29*, 364–376.

Walsh, R., & Shapiro, S. L. (2006). The meeting of meditative disciplines and western psychology: A mutually enriching dialogue. *American Psychologist, 61*(3), 227.

Weick, K. E., & Sutcliffe, K. M. (2001). Managing the unexpected.

Williams, M. J., McManus, F., Muse, K., & Williams, J. M. (2011). Mindfulness-based cognitive therapy for severe health anxiety (hypochondriasis): An interpretative phenomenological analysis of patients' experiences. *British Journal of Clinical Psychology, 50*, 379–397.

Zeidan, F., Johnson, S. K., Diamond, B. J., David, Z., & Goolkasian, P. (2010). Mindfulness meditation improves cognition: Evidence of brief mental training. *Consciousness and Cognition, 19*(2), 597–605.

Appendix

Answer these questions according to the below defined scores

1	2	3	4	5	6
Almost always	Very frequently	Somewhat frequently	Somewhat infrequently	Very infrequently	Almost never

Please tick ( ) or circle around the score

1	I could be experiencing some emotion and not be conscious of it until sometime later	1	2	3	4	5	6
2	I break or spill things because of carelessness, not paying attention, or thinking of something else	1	2	3	4	5	6
3	I find it difficult to stay focused on what's happening in the present	1	2	3	4	5	6
4	I tend to walk quickly to get where I'm going without paying attention to what I experience along the way	1	2	3	4	5	6
5	I tend not to notice feelings of physical tension or discomfort until they really grab my attention	1	2	3	4	5	6
6	I forget a person's name almost as soon as I've been told it for the first time	1	2	3	4	5	6
7	It seems I am "running on automatic", without much awareness of what I'm doing	1	2	3	4	5	6
8	I rush through activities without being really attentive to them	1	2	3	4	5	6
9	I get so focused on the goal I want to achieve that I lose touch with what I'm doing right now to get there	1	2	3	4	5	6
10	I do jobs or tasks automatically, without being aware of what I'm doing	1	2	3	4	5	6
11	I find myself listening to someone with one ear, doing something else at the same time	1	2	3	4	5	6
12	I drive places on "automatic pilot" and then wonder why I went there	1	2	3	4	5	6
13	I find myself preoccupied with the future or the past	1	2	3	4	5	6
14	I find myself doing things without paying attention	1	2	3	4	5	6
15	I snack without being aware that I'm eating	1	2	3	4	5	6

A. Ahmadi, *Mindfulness Among Students*, SpringerBriefs in Well-Being and Quality of Life Research, DOI 10.1007/978-981-10-2781-9

FSC
www.fsc.org
MIX
Papier | Fördert gute Waldnutzung
FSC® C083411

Kolibri 360 GmbH
Ferdinand-Jühlke-Straße 7
99095 Erfurt, Deutschland
produktsicherheit@kolibri360.de